Mastering Tung Acupuncture

Distal Imaging For Fast Pain Relief

Published by: Draycott Publishing

Draycott Publishing, LLC

ISBN-13:978-1-940146-06-5

MASTERING TUNG ACUPUNCTURE

DISTAL IMAGING FOR FAST PAIN RELIEF

BRAD WHISNANT, L.AC., D.A.O.M.
DEBORAH BLEECKER, L.AC., M.S.O.M.

Disclaimer

This book is designed to provide information about the subject matter covered. It is sold with the understanding that the publisher and authors are not engaged in rendering medical or other professional services. If medical or other expert assistance is required, the services of a competent professional should be sought.

Every effort has been made to make this book as complete and as accurate as possible. However, there may be mistakes both typographical and in content. Therefore, this text should be used only as a general guide and not as the ultimate source of information.

The purpose of this manual is to educate and entertain. The authors and Draycott Publishing, LLC shall have neither liability nor responsibility to any person or entity with respect to any loss or damage caused, or alleged to be caused directly or indirectly by the information contained in this book.

ACKNOWLEDGEMENTS

This book is only possible because of all the people who helped me and spent time with me. I always say, "I am not that smart. I just know really smart people."

I am grateful to Dr. Tan. I took many of his classes and followed him in his clinic. He has been very generous with his time. Without him, "distal" acupuncture would not be well known. Because of his tireless efforts over thirty years, we are able to learn this type of acupuncture, for which we are all thankful.

Dr. Wei Chieh Young has been so generous in his teachings. I can honestly say that although I have put this book together, without either of these two masters, I would not have been able to write this book.

It is because of these two individuals that so many of us have success in our clinics and are able to help others. I am grateful that I was lucky enough to spend time with these doctors.

Elotus and Evergreen herbs have been so supportive over the years with their knowledge, support, and friendship. I would say, too, that there are many others to whom I am grateful. I have had many dark days and have floundered in this medicine. I was lost and almost quit many times. I am thankful for all of you.

Last but not least, to "Cole." He was the doctor who inserted a needle into Ling gu, on my hand, which magically made my low back pain disappear. I can still remember my back pain melting away instantly. At that moment, I knew Tung acupuncture was for me. Cole educated me and let me listen to and watch him. He took me in and taught me so much. So much of what I have learned came from that original seed of Cole's friendship and knowledge.

Thank you.

When you get into a tight place and everything goes against you, till it seems as though you could not hang on a minute longer, never give up then, for that is just the place and time that the tide will turn.

Harriet Beecher Stowe

CONTENTS

Introduction

I have chosen to use the IMRs (images, mirrors, and relationships) that Dr. Wei Chieh Young and Dr. Richard Tan use in their classes.

There were obviously other influences and teachers, and I share those pearls of wisdom as well. Now, after seven years, six different countries, and 62,000 treatments, I am sharing what I have learned. All teachers have their own "take" or "flavor" for the medicine. It is my hope that you enjoy my style of "cooking."

I chose these IMRs based on my daily use of them in my own clinic and the clinical successes I have witnessed personally over the last 62,000 treatments. Are there other IMRs that you could use for these medical issues as defined by Master Tung? Yes. I also change which IMRs I use, depending on about 100 different factors. The IMRs I have chosen are based on patient comfort, ease of needling, and high clinical efficacy. I use "easy to needle," "easy to locate," and "highly dependable and successful points."

Not all of these IMRs are used *every time* on each patient. I have found in my clinic that there are a handful of IMRs and channels that work almost every time. There are "primary" IMRs that I use over 90 percent of the time (because of their dependable clinical effectiveness). There are also "secondary" IMRs that I use depending on the nature of the disease (root and branch) and the needs of the patient.

I have a saying in my clinic about Tung points. I try to use as few needles as possible, but as many as are necessary to achieve results for the patient. I do not use just one or two needles and tell the patient they are "healed." The patient needs to realize the results, not the practitioner. You will notice that many IMRs are used over and over again. I will usually use 10 percent of the IMRs 90 percent of the time. You will find this also true in your own clinic. Of your favorite points or images, 10 percent are used 90 percent of the time.

In Tung acupuncture, some of the most important and clinically effective "points" are those of zones "11.00," "22.00," "77.00," and "88.00." You will see a preponderance of these points in my choices. This is the same with the IMRs. There are those that are more clinically effective, and we decided to focus on these. This rule also applies to the channel relationships. They all work, but some relationships are much more successful in daily practice.

I usually employ a "Dao Ma" concept. Your success rate will go up when you use two to three points in a row; hence, many of my point selections are two or three points in a row. An excellent resource for further information is *Advanced Tung Style Acupuncture* by Dr. James Maher. You will also notice that if you use overlapping or redundant IMRs, your success will increase.

Most Master Tung points are treated on the opposite side, and the *most* important thing is that you obtain "de qi." If you cannot decide on "which side" the pain or internal issue is located, you can treat either side. My hope is that by treating tens of thousands of patients, and after many years of practice, each of us will see for ourselves which points or IMRs work the best for ourselves. Master Tung has given us such an amazing acupuncture system. It is through hard work, determination, and experience that we can fully understand it.

Master Tung said, "Observe for yourself, and then think about it." Master Tung never wanted any of us to blindly follow his "point selection." Master Tung never wanted any of us to blindly follow his IMRs. He wanted us to think, ponder, listen, learn, and improve. It is my hope that the IMRs and points I have suggested are a "starting point" for further elucidation to be pursued by each acupuncturist. As Buddha said, "I can show you the path, but it is you who must walk it."

CHAPTER 1

WHY DO IMAGING AND MIRRORING WORK?

The Master Tung method and/or the "distal method" is over 2,500 years old and is derived from the I-Ching, one of the oldest books in the world. This method has several names: "I-Ching Acupuncture," "The Balance Method," or "Distal Point Acupuncture." Regardless of the name, the effects are nothing less than miraculous. One of the main concepts of Master Tung acupuncture is "imaging and mirroring." We know imaging and mirroring work from a clinical perspective; this can be seen daily in the clinic. But how and why does it work?

The best example we can use to explain how imaging and mirroring work is the ear. We know in Chinese medicine that hearing loss, especially age-related hearing loss, can be due to kidney weakness, jing loss, or kidney yin and/or yang issues. It can be other TCM pathologies, of course, but let us just assume it is the kidney (some pathology of TCM kidney issues). This is by far the most common type of hearing loss we see.

If we go to any doctor and tell them hearing loss is due to a kidney deficiency, most will laugh us out of their office. If we tell our patients that we need to treat their kidneys to heal their ears, they are likely to look confused. This, though, is not that far from the truth.

The kidney and ear, via embryology, are the only two tissues that at one point were the same. In Chinese medicine, what is another name for the ear? It is called the outer kidney. Why is this? Is it some hookie-dookie mystical, crazy Chinese medicine? The kidney and ear were *once the same tissue.*

During development of the kidney, the tissue "breaks apart." One part moves to your back and becomes your kidney. The other part of this tissue migrates to your head and becomes your ear. It is amazing that our ancestors already knew this thousands of years ago.

It is interesting to note. How do Western doctors and other Western-minded practitioners treat age-related hearing loss? Typically, they have no answer. The few who are current on their research have recently been prescribing or suggesting the supplement called the "hearing hormone." This hormone is called Aldosterone. Can you guess where it is made? Aldosterone is made in the adrenal glands.

The Chinese were 95 percent correct on anatomy in 2000 BC. The only thing they did not "separate" out were the endocrine glands. When we treat the kidneys, we are also treating the adrenal glands.

The adrenal glands are endocrine glands, and they are located on the top of the kidneys. When Chinese medicine refers to the kidneys, they are including the adrenals. In Chinese medicine, most would agree that, when it comes to pulse diagnosis, there are two kidney pulses. The right pulse pertains to the "western kidney." This is the actual function of the kidney—filtration, water metabolism, etc.

The left-side kidney pulse is known as the "Chinese kidney pulse." This pulse is typically associated with strength, energy, libido, and reproduction. This pulse represents the adrenal glands and the adrenal function of the kidneys. Though they are separate in Western medicine, they were originally grouped together in Chinese medicine.

So 3,000 years ago the ancients knew that if we stimulate the kidney (i.e., the adrenal and kidney), we can release aldosterone into our bloodstream and thus improve hearing. There are numerous research studies on the effects of aldosterone and age-related hearing loss.

So what does this have to do with image, mirror, and tissue relationships? This helps us understand why it makes sense that the elbow can fix the knee. Or that the foot can fix the face. Or that the lungs are on the biceps, and the heart is on the upper thigh. This helps explain the numerous images and mirrors. Our body is a connected organism. Though you and I may see different "pieces" of our body—an arm, a foot, a face, an ear, or a kidney—it is all related. Our body is a system—a physical, emotional, and spiritual system. When we influence one piece, we cause a reaction on another piece somewhere else. This is what the ancients realized.

As an embryo, we are all one cell. From a zygote, we became a polygote and then four cells, eight cells, sixteen cells, etc., until we eventually become a full-fledged 100 trillion–cell human being. This is important because all the genetic information from that one cell is in all 100 trillion cells in our body.

Granted, the cells are different, but the DNA, the genetic material, is the same in all the cells. Hence, we have the yin/yang theory of the yin within the yang, and the yang within the yin. The micro in the macro, the universe in the human, and the human in the universe.

As we developed, our cells were a tube, in rudimentary terms. As this tube split in two, we had two parts. As the two parts separated again, we had a top and bottom, although visually we see up and down or left and right. For the brain, the same neural connections that are in the left are in the right (they came from each other). The same neural connections are in the top and bottom (they came from each other). The same neural connections in the left, right, up, and down are *all the same*. They all came from each other.

This is why the human body can be treated in so many places. We can find images and mirrors all over, but the whole human body is also represented in the sole of foot, the hand, the ear, the head, any bone, any finger, and any toe. The body representations are endless. This is why distal acupuncture works.

You and I see a left and right, or a leg bone and an arm bone. The body certainly sees this as well, but it also sees the other as identical. It is like looking at your child as an adult. Your son or daughter might be fully grown, and you see that, but you can also still see the child in them.

We see this in parents and their children. How many children act like their parents? How many smile like their parents? It is not the same, but it is. This is similar to the theory of images and mirrors on the body. We see different things visually, but the brain has a different visual representation of the human body. If you see a picture of what the brain "sees," you will see a different-looking human.

The brain sees you and me with a huge head, huge lips, huge eyes, huge nose, and a huge mouth. It sees a super small chest, back, upper arms, and abdomen. It sees a huge genital area, huge lower arms, even bigger hands, and even bigger fingers. It sees the upper legs as small and the lower legs as huge. It sees the lower legs as bigger, and the foot and toes bigger and bigger. For more detailed information on this, see the book *Mapping the Mind* by Rita Carter.

13

Why is this important? The fact that the brain sees larger or smaller parts of the body is the representation of the neural density in the brain. So speaking in simple terms, since the brain sees the lower limbs (both arms and legs) as "larger," a needle placed in the lower limbs will cause a larger reaction in the brain. This larger reaction will cause more effects. The stronger the effects, the greater the healing. Or we can needle tissue that is not as dense with nerves. This will typically cause a smaller reaction in the brain, which will reduce the effects and slow the healing.

One of the categories of acupuncture points is called the "transport points." Similar to understanding algebra in order to understand chemistry, the transport points are a foundational step to higher learning in Chinese medicine.

The five transporting (shu) points are referred to as follows: Jing (Well), Ying (Spring), Shu (Stream), Jing (River), and He (Sea). These acupuncture points belong to the "twelve regular" meridians and are located below the elbows or knees. The five transporting (Shu) points start at the tip of the four limbs and continue all the way to the elbows or knees.

Each transport point will have a general definition that includes information on how the Qi flows at the transport point and some general pathology. The movement of Qi is correlated with the movement of water. At the Jing Well point, Qi emanates like a well. The Ying Spring point is the point where Qi glides. The Shu Stream point is the point where Qi flows through. The Jing River point is where Qi flows. The He Sea point is where the rivers join the sea.

So why are the transport points located in the area from the elbows to fingers, and the knees to toes? I do not think it is by chance. Why are they not from the shoulders to elbows, and the knees to hips? The proverbial river of qi could start anywhere or go anywhere, so why is it where it is? Part of the answer is that the more distal we get on the extremities, the higher density of nerves we have. The higher density of nerves we have, the higher the stimulus that is created by the needle in the mid cortex of the brain. The more the mid cortex is stimulated (remember the most important thing in Tung acupuncture is to obtain De qi), the faster the healing will occur.

When it comes to distal acupuncture, you will see in the clinic that the more distal you get from the injury, the better your outcome will be. Why is it that in Master

Tung acupuncture, the points 77.01-2-3 are on the ankle? These points treat the neck. The same tissue, bones, muscles, and channels that balance the neck can be found in the lower arm. So why are these powerful points in the ankle and not the wrist?

In my opinion, Master Tung noticed that the more distal he was from the problem area, the better results he had. Even in Tan acupuncture, the main thrust of the system is to balance channels. You are to pick the right image, pick the diseased channel, and then pick a channel to heal the diseased channel.

Dr. Tan even says, "When it comes to fingers treating toes, or toes treating fingers you can forget the channels." He continues, "Just focus on the image." The image is so powerful you do not need to worry about what channel balances the affected channel. It is interesting to note that doing this, "forgetting what channels balance the other channels," can be forgone when we are dealing with the most distal extremities. On any other part of the body, you need to correctly identify the sick meridian and choose a healthy meridian to fix it.

I think this is true. It is also true that because the images are so distal to each other, the effect is so strong; that is why it works so well. In my clinic, if I have two options to treat one condition, I will always pick the most distal point(s). This is not to say local points do not work—obviously they do. I am just saying that if you are using a distal method, it is better to always pick the most distal choice.

The mapping, image, and mirror is not a theoretical concept. It is based on the anatomy and the brain. It is reliable, predictable, and consistent. Understanding this aspect takes the magic out, but it makes it much more real for our patients and us. It is also much simpler to explain that it is a "brain" thing and not a "magic" thing. If it were magic, I could cure everybody in one treatment. It is not magic, so I need to treat most patients more than one time.

You have enemies? Good. That means you have stood up for something, sometime in your life.

Winston Churchill

Success consists of going from failure to failure without loss of enthusiasm.

Winston Churchill

CHAPTER 2

IMAGING AND MIRRORING TECHNIQUES

One for One Image

In Master Tung acupuncture, one of the major theories or ideas is the idea of "image, mirrors, or segments." We will discuss the "twelve segments," and the "three jiaos." We will also discuss mirrors in detail. Another theory of Master Tung acupuncture is "images." I am sure everyone has heard of "images." There are many different "sizes" of images, but the one we need to discuss first is the "one for one image." This is probably the most commonly used image in the clinic.

As we discuss mirrors and images, rest assured that for every image I discuss, there are ten more that I do not mention. Learning Chinese medicine is a lifelong process. I do not have all the answers; nobody does. You will need to practice in real life, on real patients, and make real mistakes. You will learn; you will fail; and you will relearn, rethink, and retry. We are all *students forever*. So as we embark on our journey to understand images and mirrors, keep an open mind. Minds are like parachutes; they work only when they are open.

We said earlier that "mirrors" are something of which you have "two things" on your body. These "mirrors" look just alike. Our example was the humerus and the femur. Another mirror is the radius and the tibia, or the ulna and the fibula. We said the ulnar tendon is just like the Achilles tendon. We even said the shoulder is like the hip. These are all ideas of "mirrors." So what is our image?

Our first image is made by taking the torso and putting the whole torso on the arm or the leg. The torso does not have anything that looks just like a torso; we have only one. Therefore, we must "image" a torso somewhere. You can obviously do that in scalp, ear, or hand acupuncture.

In Master Tung acupuncture, we are going to image the whole torso on the whole arm or the whole leg. This is called a one for one image. This is one torso on one full limb (either arm or leg). I like this one for one image because clinically it is extremely reliable and effective. There are numerous Tung points that can be explained with this image. Some of the most clinically effective points and treatments I have done are from this image. Let us spend some more time on this image.

Our first step is to decide where to start. We will explain later that we can also reverse the image. Let us start with the arm. The hand is the head. The tips of the fingers are the top of the head. The knuckles (SI 3, TW 3, LI 3) area is the C1 atlas/axis. As we progress proximally on the hand, the palm (HT 8 area) is the eyes, ears, teeth, and mouth. The wrist/palm is the chin, and the wrist joint is C7/T1.

[handwritten margin note: C1 atlas/axis]

I always like to think in terms of "joints." The knuckles are your very first "joint," C1, and the wrist is the second joint on your spine, C7/T1. For me, checking my "joints" always keeps me on track with my image. Following your "joints" is important. If you are trying to image the face, it is obviously in between the head and neck. So our image must be in between the knuckles and the wrist. Watching your joints will help you find your way if you get lost.

From the wrist, moving proximally, we are moving up the arm in the direction of the shoulder. This would image us moving inferiorly down the spine. TW 5-6-7 would represent the zone of T4-5-6-7. The elbow represents the belly button, on the same line as L2. From the elbow, we continue to move proximally up the arm. The mid upper arm is the area of L3-4. The shoulder joint is L5/S1, with the top of the shoulder, the acromion, in the S1-4 area.

Though I am suggesting that the image here lines up with the joint at C1 or C7/T1 or L2 or L5, this does not mean it images only the dorsal side of the body. Any time we find a certain landmark on our image, I want you to visualize it in your mind; in this instance, the elbow is the belly button. That "image" is a circumference. So what else is on the same "line" as the belly button, the lower ribs, the liver, L2, etc.?

The wrist is a much better image for L5/S1 versus "just the lower arm" because the joints on this image do not match up. What looks more like a homologous structure, the lower arm or the actual joint (the wrist joint) of the lower arm? The actual joint of the wrist is/treats the L5/S1 joint, or low back pain, versus the lower mid arm, which is a poor homologous relationship.

Then, using the same height theory, this will change depending on the arm length of the individual. It does not always work if the patient has short or long arms. With this theory, the L5/S1 joint is usually around the lower arm, not the joint space of the wrist.

Without a doubt, it will still work, but again, we are interested in the "best" images and the most "reliable" images, day in and day out in our clinic. I clinically prefer to "watch my lines and levels" but also, more importantly, not to lose sight of the joints and images presented by Master Tung and Dr. Tan.

Always remember, any "spot" we image has a circle around it. This is similar to how HT 8 images the head, in particular the eyes. If we draw a line around the head, that HT 8 spot will image the eyes, the temporal side of the head, and the occipital protuberance. The question is, "Does it treat all that?" Obviously, the answer is "no." We have to decide on our channel, our diagnosis, and many other factors before we decide on treatment points. Finding the correct image is the *first step* in choosing appropriate treatment points.

Acromion	Shoulder girdle, S2-3-4
Ball-and-socket joint of the shoulder	L5/S1
Belly button	L2
Fingers	Top of head
Heart area	Eyes
Knuckles	C1/axis/atlas
Lower arm	Upper neck
Mid lower arm	Mid upper back
Mid upper arm	L3-4
Palm of hand	Chin
Wrist	C7/T1

Joints

This entire image, as you will hear time and time again, can be reversed. The acromion is the top of the head. The shoulder joint is C1 axis and atlas. The shoulder muscles are the face, and where the deltoid muscles attach to the humerus is the chin. The mid upper back is the upper arm, and the belly button is the elbow. Mid lower arm is the L3-4, and the wrist joint is L5/S1 joint. The hand and fingers are the sacrum/coccyx.

Elbow joint	L2
Knuckles of hand	C1
Shoulder joint	L5/S1
Wrist joint	C7/T1

Both of these images work, of course. Which image do you think is more reliable and effective? The first image we discussed is much more effective and reliable. The hand acts and looks much like the face. The head pivots on the C7/T1 joint, and so does the hand. The hand pivots at the wrist. If we reverse it, the image really is a muscle attachment of the lateral deltoid. That is very similar to how our head acts. Noticing these relationships and finding the most consistent ones will affect your clinic in a positive way.

Let us see if any of the Tung points matches this definition of our one torso for one upper limb image. The point 22.04, Da bai/LI 3 is wonderful for headaches. We just said the knuckles are the C1 axis/atlas. If we draw a circle around the head, many patients have headaches in that area.

The points 33.01-2-3 are on the LI channel, very close to LI 5-6-7 (different locations, of course). Though these points are famous for treating gynecological problems, they are also clinically effective for treating throat issues. We just said that the wrist joint was C7/T1, so if we are just proximal to the wrist, we are then just inferior to the superior aspect of the throat. We also said you can reverse the image, and that the wrist was L5/S1.

If we are super proximal to the wrist joint, then we are just superior to the L5/S1 juncture. The points 33.01-2-3 are used most often for gynecological issues. The image explains both of these uses quite well. There are many upper arm Tung points, 44.02-3 in particular, that treat low back pain.

We said that the elbow was L2. The points 44.02 and 44.03 are just proximal to the elbow joints. If we are just proximal to the elbow joint, then we are just inferior to the L2 area. These points, 44.02-3, are also great for upper thoracic pain. If we reverse the image, the elbow is the L2 juncture. If the head is the shoulder, then the area just proximal to the elbow is L2, and moving superior on the spine. These 44.02-3 points treat T8-12 area. Again, both uses of these points are explained via our image of one torso for one limb.

This image can also be placed on the leg. We can place a full torso on the full leg, and we can, as always, reverse it. Since the leg is a mirror of the arm, the leg and its "joints" and image will be much the same. The tips of the toes are the top of the head. The knuckles of the foot are the C1 atlas/axis. The ankle is the C7/T1. The upper back is imaged as the lower leg. The knee is the belly button. The mid upper thigh is the L3-4; the lower abdomen area and the hip joint are the L5/S1 joints, with the pelvis being the S2-3-4.

This image can also be reversed. The pelvis is at the top, with the hip being the head. The ball-and-socket joint of the hip is the C1 axis/atlas. The C7/T1 is just distal to the ball-and-socket joint of the hip. The upper thigh is the upper thoracic of the back. The knee is the belly button. The lower leg is the lower abdomen and L3-4 area. The ankle joint is the L5/S1 joint, and the foot and toes are the sacrum S2-3-4.

Are there Master Tung points on the lower leg that can help us see this image? Of course there are! Men jin or 66.05, which is just proximal to ST 43, is used for headaches, and it is also used for uterus issues. Via our image of one full torso for one full limb, the foot is either the head or the groin area.

The image is perfect. The point 77.21, which is very close to SP 6, is used for "lower" back pain. Here, with our image of the full torso on the full leg with the hip being the head, the knee being the belly button, and the ankle being L5/S1, we can see how the SP 6 area is the lower back, L2-3-4-5 zone.

We can look at 88.01-2-3, which is important for hearing issues. These points are on the mid upper thigh. If our image is the hip as the head and the knee as the belly button, then where is the heart? The heart is about halfway between the head and the belly button, and the points are halfway on the upper thigh.

Toe knuckles	C1
Ankle	C7/T1
Knee	L2
Hip	L5, S1
Pelvic girdle	S2-3-4

And ...

Hip joint	C1, axis/atlas
3 cun distally	C7, T1, (There is no joint, which is why I do not like this image.)
Knee	L2
Ankle	L5/S1
Toes	S2-3-4

Again, just like the upper arm, I do not like to reverse this image as much because the "joints" do not line up when we reverse it. It is not as homologous as the foot and head image. They both still work, but in my opinion it is usually more clinically effective to use the hand as the head, the ankle as C7/T1, and the lower leg as the upper back. The knee is L2, the belly button is the mid upper thigh. The lower back and hip joint are L5/S1.

There is one more image that I want to discuss, the image made using the full torso on the full limb. This idea will change the location of the previous images. I think it is important to discuss both because they are both applicable. This is the image of the "same level."

The "same level" means that we look at the torso and look at the arm. We see a spot on the torso, and then we take that *exact* same height and transfer it over to the arm. So if we look at the chest and want to treat the chest, we look at the arm. In this case, the upper arm then lines up with the chest.

According to our theory, that is the correct image to use where the torso and the arm line up. If we look at the heart, the heart and middle deltoid are at the same level. This theory says that in order to treat the heart, we would consider treating the shoulder. Interesting enough, 44.06, jian zhong, is in the middle of the deltoid muscle, and it treats the heart.

If we wanted to treat the lower intestines, we would look at the torso and see with which part of the arm it lines up. The lower intestines are a match for the lower arm. The point 33.10, which is called intestine gate in Tung acupuncture, is not surprisingly used for digestive complaints.

This theory also says that you can take the same spot you found on the arm and transfer that same spot to the leg. Therefore, in our case of 33.10, the lower arm treats the lower intestines. We can take that *exact* spot, move it to the leg, and treat that spot. This works. The points 77.24-25 are on the lower leg, and they treat digestive complaints.

Both of these Master Tung theories are used a lot, and both have shortcomings. It can get confusing for some when they see the elbow as L2 and the wrist as L5. It stands to reason that the length between the lower and upper arm are the same. When we image it, however, the upper arm covers the length of head to the belly button, *but* the area from the elbow to the wrist (basically the same length from the shoulder to the elbow) now covers only the belly button to the groin. The belly button to the groin is a much shorter distance than the head to the belly button. However, the distances from the shoulder to elbow, and the elbow to groin are much shorter. It does not make perfect sense.

Theories help explain points. They help us rationalize why we are choosing our points. However, as always, clinical experience will prove if we chose the correct points.

Twelve Segments

Any bone can be broken down into twelve segments. Why is LI 11 so great for dizziness? LI 11 is the "head." The radius is broken down into twelve equal segments: head, neck, upper limbs, lungs/heart, liver, stomach, duodenum, kidney, low back, lower limbs, thigh, and foot.

Just like the three jiaos, any bone can be broken down further from three segments of the upper, middle, and lower jiao into twelve segments. The first questions I asked are: Where do these twelve segments come from? Why are there twelve and not eleven or thirteen? When they say "upper limbs" does that mean the bicep or the tricep? What part of the bicep, the big head or the smaller head? What part of the stomach? And why the duodenum and not the jejunum?

I think this is a very Western way of thinking. We want specifics, when we need to trust the body and the thinking of the ancient scholars. There is much theory and history as to why they came up with twelve segments and why each segment correlated to a particular body part. However, these points treat each of these parts in general terms. Recently I had a patient with heart palpations. I used the 4 point in the twelve segments, "heart and lungs," for her heart. I used other points as well, but one of images I used was the twelve segments.

I have clinically accepted the twelve segments as such and put them to the test over the years. I have needled all twelve segments on each bone to give a patient a "total body treatment." The results, though twelve needles is a lot, have always been wonderful. I have at times also treated just the "liver, stomach, duodenum, and kidney" points for generalized middle jiao discomfort, and they are very effective.

Maybe just low back pain was the "kidney, low back, low limbs, thigh, and foot points." Again, that is a few too many points, but I still get great results. The twelve segments is certainly a viable theory and clinically effective no matter where or how you use it.

The most popular bone is the second metacarpal bone. Another example of this is the thigh bone, or the femur. The bone is broken down into twelve equidistant points. The first point is found just as you fall off distally at the head of the femur. If we were using the second metacarpal point, LI 3 would be the head. There is a secret point just a few fen proximal to LI 3. This is a point for insomnia. There is no secret to it. The point is at the ninth segment of the twelve segments, the heart/lungs. When we understand the theory, it sheds light on the "secrets."

Here is why Da bai, 22.04, is so famous for headaches in Master Tung acupuncture. One theory says it is the upper jiao, but here is a more specialized theory. According to the twelve segments theory, in that upper jiao, LI 3, or the first point in our twelve-point segment, is the head. What part of the head? We do not know this just by using this theory. We would have to apply channel theory or additional relationships from the Tung acupuncture system.

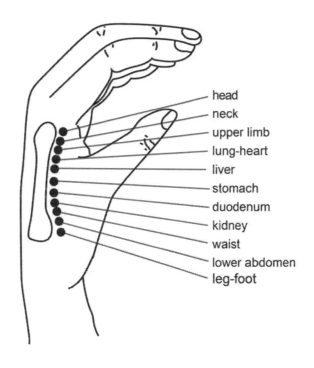

As always, the twelve segments can be reversed. Now the "head" would be at the base of the second metacarpal joint, and the "foot" would be LI 3 or Da bai. There are two very popular points in Master Tung acupuncture, 22.01-02 double saint and double child. They are located on the thenar eminence, close to the area of LU 10.

The most proximal thumb bone is broken into three equidistant sections. Two pins are placed equidistant from each other. It is interesting to note that these points treat upper neck pain. If we apply the twelve segments to this theory, we find that points correspond with the head, neck, and upper limbs area.

If we reverse it, the other points will line up with the same three points—"head, neck, and upper limbs." There are other theories as to why these points are effective, but explaining them or seeing every bone as a twelve-segment bone is of great importance.

When we look at the tissue, we should look not at where to put the needles, the micro picture, but first at the macro picture. There are three parts to this tissue. Within those three parts, we can further divide it into twelve segments. Those three jiaos and twelve segments can all be reversed. Why is LI 11 so great for head pain or dizziness? The dizziness can be explained from a five-element perspective, and also by the five antique, with the wood helping the liver and tendons to reduce shaking.

From a twelve-segment Master Tung perspective, LI 11 is at the most proximal end of the radius. It is the "first point" in the twelve segments. It can be either the upper jiao or the lower jiao, the "head or the foot." LI 11 is great for generalized head and upper jiao issues.

The point LI 4, Hegu, though not a Master Tung point, can be used for digestion problems. (See Dr. Tan's "magical 8 or 9 for digestion). Here, LI 4 is in the middle of the twelve segments and in the middle jiao. The middle segment of twelve segments is the stomach.

The point KD 7 in TCM is used to tonify the kidneys. If we break down the tibia into twelve segments and move over the kidney channel, KD 7 is right about where the seventh and eigth segment is; this is the low back and kidney.

It is interesting to note that there are twelve segments with three jiaos. So each jiao receives four points. The upper jiao would be the head, neck, upper limbs, and lungs. The middle jiao, or segments 5 through 8, are the liver, stomach, duodenum, and kidney. The lower jiao, or the 9-12 segments, are the low back, lower limbs, thigh, and foot.

We can break down the tibia into twelve segments. The point 77.08 is basically ST 36. This is right at the segment of the head as per the twelve segments. This point is also very effective for headaches.

As with any theory or point, we ask if this is the only reason why or why not points "work." The answer is of course not. This twelve-segment theory gives us insights. When looking at a point, we need to take a step back and realize what other theories are at play. The biggest concept we have to grasp here is that the whole body can be treated via the twelve segments. The twelve segments allow us to treat specifically twelve points on the body, on any bone, anywhere on the body.

Fully Clothed Acupuncture

(The Arm Can Treat the Arm, the Arm Can Treat the Leg)

The arm can treat the arm, and the arm can treat the leg. We already know from a mirroring concept that the leg treats the arm, and the arm treats the leg. There is no better example than San cha san, A02. It is inserted at TW 2 and ends at the base of the fourth and fifth metacarpal. This point is one of the ten most popular points in Master Tung acupuncture.

In this example, San cha san treats same side shoulder pain. San cha san is on the TW channel, and it treats TW shoulder pain. The channel we are using here, in this case the TW, always treats itself. Therefore, TW treats TW on the same side. The fingers and wrist treat the shoulder. This is because the end of the arm (the fingers) treats the start of the arm (the shoulder). This is very similar to the theory of the first point on the channel treating the last point in the channel.

This is also similar because you can take an image and reverse it. If we can take any image and reverse it, then does it not make sense that the wrist and fingers would treat the shoulder? We frequently use the arm to treat the leg, do we not? We also say you can reverse the image of the arm to treat the leg. Therefore, it makes sense that the arm can treat itself. The wrist/fingers and the shoulder are images of each other. So we know the arm can treat itself.

The arm can also treat the other arm. The wrist treats the opposite shoulder, the elbow treats the elbow, and the shoulder treats the wrist. Fan hou jue is a Tung point with no number, but it is on the thumb. This point treats opposite-side shoulder pain, and quite frankly, it does so remarkably. It is always my first choice for opposite-arm shoulder pain. I will needle Fan hou jue on the thumb, treating the opposite shoulder. I will then add in same side San cha san, which is the same side wrist treating same side shoulder.

These two points will usually take away 90–100 percent of the shoulder pain. Fan hou jue is such a remarkable point. It balances and/or treats the complete shoulder; it is not "channel" specific. That is how powerful it is. The addition of San cha san is the theory using a "guide" for your treatment. That theory will be for another book; it is not about images or mirrors.

In the same way that the lower arm can treat the upper arm, and the upper arm can treat the lower arm, the lower leg can treat the upper leg. The three lateral passes are equally distributed on the lower leg. They help with any type of systemic pain, among many other things. I often use these three points to treat same side upper leg problems. Again, these points on the lower leg treat the upper leg, but they are channel specific.

Step 1 is always choosing the right image or mirror. Step 2 is figuring out what channel you are treating. This will guide what channel you need to use as your healing channel. This is how the famous Dr. Tan teaches: Find your sick meridian. Pick the meridian that will fix that diseased meridian. Step 3 is picking the correct image or mirror. I suggest all readers continue their education with Dr. Tan classes and books. His teachings are remarkable.

I want to return to the three lateral passes and lower leg. These points are on the GB meridian. I usually do not have my patients undress. If they have upper leg pain on the GB channel, my first choice would be the upper arm to treat it. They are both the same structure.

If the patient is wearing long sleeves and pants, how can I treat her? My favorite homologous images are not available. If my patient has right hand pain, the best choice would be the left foot. However, just last month I treated a Vietnam veteran. He had only a right leg. He lost his left foot in the war. What can I do now? This theory of arm for arm or leg for leg comes into play.

We can use the lower portion of the same side leg to treat the upper portion of the same side leg. We could indeed use the upper portion of the leg to treat the lower portion of the same leg. The ankle of the same leg will treat the hip of the same leg. I frequently use GB 40 to treat GB hip pain. The hip of the same leg can treat the ankle of the same leg.

Any leg can be used to treat the opposite leg. The right side ankle can treat the left side hip, or vice versa. The right side ankle can treat the left side ankle, or vice versa. The right side hip can treat the left side ankle or vice versa. The right side hip can treat the left side hip or vice versa. There is also a choice with imaging and mirroring.

Ankle	Hip
Ankle, right side	Ankle, left side
Hip	Ankle
Hip, right side	Ankle, left side
Leg	Opposite leg
Leg, lower area	Leg, upper area, same side

The GB 40 point is a great example of this. I will often insert a needle in the ankle to treat the hip joint. The ankle joint looks much like the hip joint. One of the most valuable treatment points for hip pain is to insert a needle around the lateral malleolus. The lateral anklebone is the bottom of foot, treating the same side hip pain. The bottom of the leg is used to treat the top of the leg. If I were to choose different channels, we could also use the ankle to treat opposite hip pain very successfully.

Best hip pain treatment = Lateral malleolus

There is one more theory with arm for arm or leg for leg. I call it the same spot treatment. It is not my treatment. It is a Master Tung theory. I was once taught the

Distal Imaging

easiest way to do Tung acupuncture was to "just to find the exact spot of pain on the opposite limb and needle that spot, and then add in GB 31 or 88.25 on the same side." In Tung acupuncture, GB 31 or 88.25 is the best point for insomnia, stress, and overall systemic pain regardless of its location. It is a top-ten point and therapeutically irreplaceable.

No matter where the pain is, just find that same spot on the other same limb, needle it, and then add in 88.25. The point 88.25 becomes the "guide point" or the supporting point for the treatment.

This theory works, and when you are confused, lost, or do not know where to start, you can use this. I find much better results using different images, but this image of same for same spot does work. It is quick, it is effective, and it works consistently. I have used this a lot when I treat overseas.

For example, last year I was in Vietnam treating people for free. I was treating 150 people a day. Needless to say, once we had interviewed them and I knew what my treatment plan was, I would treat very quickly. This type of treatment is a quick and effective way to treat. Make no mistake about it though, it is "not just a quick way to treat." It is backed by current research.

The current research shows that when a needle is inserted in LI 4 (or any spot for that matter), the *exact* same spot is vasodilated, blood enriched, and nutrient enriched; receives painkillers; experiences a reduction in tissue inflammation and relaxation of nerves/muscles; and new tissue is created in that mirror spot.

It is so interesting that after 3,000 years, modern research proves our theories correct. A great example that I see a lot in the clinic is low back pain and knee pain. I can needle BL 40 for the same side back pain (BL will fix BL same side, and opposite KD) in this case, left-sided back pain. I needle the left side BL 40. I then tell my patient to breathe and ask her how it is now. The pain will most likely be gone. The interesting thing is, if that patient also had knee pain on the right, at any part of the BL channel area, her knee pain will also be gone. I see a lot of people with knee and back pain, so I often see this happen in my clinic.

Another common example is headaches, and patients with hand pain. I can insert needles for the headache on the same side. Let us say they have TW and LI channel headaches, or yang ming or shao yang headaches. They have heat, inflammation, and other liver imbalances. Regardless of the theory, LI 3 and TW 3 (Da bai and San cha san) are the correct choices. The hand images the face, and via channel theory, the same channel is treated on the same side. These two points will treat and cure the same side headaches that are on the TW and LI channels in the face. The points were inserted on the right hand, and they treated the right side of the face.

In addition, let us say this patient *also* had left sided lateral head pain. The needles that were inserted on the right hand will treat the left side of face. The wrist can image the head. Almost all points are treated on the opposite side, except when the same channel is treating itself. In this case, TW and LI were chosen. Therefore, TW and LI will treat and fix opposite side GB and ST pain. So with our two points in the right hand, we treated not only the right side, but also the left side of the face. Here is where it gets interesting.

Let us say this patient also happened to have left-sided hand pain. The needles inserted on the right hand, LI 3/ Da bai and San cha san, basically TW 3, treated the SAME spot on the left hand.

The important thing to understand with this theory is that there are many things happening all over the body when we insert a needle in any location. As our understanding grows and deepens, this is how we can reduce the number of needles we use. We can see the vast theories that are applicable before we insert a needle. As we insert one, two, three, or four needles, we can see that we are treating so many conditions, so many places, so many images all at the same time.

Face on Leg or Arm

A very important image to discuss is the face. The face can be imaged on the full leg or the full arm. This term is (or could be) called a full-face image, on a full-limb image. This is important because clinically, it is an image I use very often. It is extremely effective and very reliable.

We have talked about other images for the face. The torso was imaged on the arm and/or leg, which meant the face was on the hand or foot, and the top of the head was the fingers or toes. It meant the chin was the wrist or the ankle. We also said we could image the whole torso on the limb in a reversed fashion.

This would mean that the top of the head was the top of the shoulder, or the top of the hip, and the nose was mid deltoid or mid upper hip. The chin, then, was just below the mid deltoid and/or just below mid-thigh.

We can also image the torso (which includes the head and face) on the toes and fingers, as well as on the head and the ear. There are many places to image the face.

The new image I would like to discuss, and one that has great clinical applications, is the face being represented on a limb. This means the whole face, from the top of the head to the chin, is imaged on either the full arm or full leg.

Chin	Ankle
Eyes and ears	Knee area
Hip	Head
Nose	ST 36 proximal
Toes	Bottom of the chin
Upper thigh	Forehead

Of course, both of these images could be reversed, but you will find that most of the clinical applications are around the *knee* or *elbow* area, so reversing the image is somewhat of a moot point. No matter how we reverse it, the knee or elbow area is somewhat the same.

These are some of my favorite points around this area for clinical applications. We have discussed HT 8 for headaches, which is effective because you can put the whole torso on the arm. That being said, the hand was the head, and HT 8 location was the level of the eyes.

Gall Bladder Meridian Headaches

A better and more clinically effective point to use is about one cun distal to HT 3. I have yet to see a point that matches the clinical effectiveness of this point for GB meridian headaches. This point is what I call HT 3.20.

The best part of this distal HT 3 is that it is much less painful than HT 8 for my patients. I also think the structure is better at HT 3 versus HT 8. In my opinion, most headaches are usually inflammatory or constrictive in nature.

There are forty-three muscles in your face. Depending on how you group the head and neck muscles, you could say there are over sixty muscles in the face. A headache is often caused by inflammation. Trauma or tight muscles restrict proper blood flow. The structure of HT 3 is better than HT 8. There is a bigger muscle at HT 3 versus HT 8. There is a bigger artery at HT 3 versus HT 8. We know from "like for like" and "tissue for tissue" that the better correspondence of not only the point but also the tissue will improve our outcome. This is why, I think, a distal HT 3 is so much better.

Stuffy Nose

I frequently use a distal PC 3 about one cun from the traditional PC 3. It is an amazing point for stuffy nose. The hand jue yin balances the foot yang ming. The image of the full face on the full arm is at work here. The nose is just below the elbow. The PC 3 balances and treats the ST. It is a very effective point, though no named point is located there.

I share these examples because these are points that are "made up" based on theory. They are tested in the clinic. We hypothesize, "Based on this theory, this point should work." This is much the same way they discovered these points and theories 3,000 years ago. They probably thought: Let us needle this because our theory says it should work. Now let us see if it works when we use it on over 10,000 patients with the same condition. If it does, we will keep it. If it does not, we will get rid of it.

Depression

The leg has even greater implications. Recent research shows GB 34 is beneficial for depression. It does not really make sense until we are able to see that GB 34 is the image of the head, where depression is located. The face can be imaged on the leg. GB 34 is the mid head, right on the same level of the pineal gland. The pineal gland is what is responsible for our "happy chemicals."

Some very famous Tung points, 77.22-23, are magnificent for headache on the GB and ST meridians as well as for teeth and jaw pain. It is a two-point unit. One point is around ST 36, between the ST and GB meridians (the headache indications), and the next point is 2 cun distal (the teeth applications). That two-point unit never ceases to amaze me.

From the full face being on a full leg, we can see these points are a few cun below the patella. A few cun below the patella are the head and teeth. You might say, "I am too low for the head. You said the eyes were the knee. If we go below the knee, are we not going down the face? If we are below the knee, we must be imaging the nose or teeth, but not the head." You are correct. However, remember, we can *reverse it.*

So now, the head is at the toes, the eyes are the knees, and the chin is the hip. Seeing this imaged both ways, reversed and not reversed, shows us we are treating a few cun above and below the eyes. A few cun above and below the eyes includes the forehead, eyebrows, eyes, cheekbones, teeth, and nose. These points, 77.22-23, treat all of those indications.

Headaches

[handwritten: ST 36, 4.5 cun distal]

Tung points 77.08 and 77.09 treat many things. The point 77.08 is one of the most frequently used Tung points. One of the indications is for headaches. The image is perfect. With the full face on the leg, the eyes are right at the knee. TCM even references ST 35 as right around the "eyes of the knee."

[handwritten: GB 31]

The point 88.25 is one of the top ten most frequently used points by Master Tung. It is most famous for its ability to treat overall pain, but in particular its remarkable ability for headache pain. With this image we can see why: the mid-thigh is the forehead, where most headaches are. If we reverse the image, it is also the lower face. So this point treats the upper mid head and lower mid head when we image the full face on the full leg.

Sinus Problems

The Si mas, points 88.17-18-19, are one of the most famous Dao Mas of Master Tung. These points are very famous for all sinus issues. If the eyes are the knee, where would the nose be? If we reverse the image, the forehead is the feet. The knees are the eyes, and just below the eyes is the nose. Well, just proximal to the knee are the points 88.17-18-19. Yes, there are about fifteen other reasons why these points work, but you can see the image is perfect.

I will frequently use the hand image of the head and the head image of the elbow together. This covers both images and "doubles up my images," a very effective technique. Granted, it is a few more needles, but it is super effective.

If you were to use TCM points, your point selections might look like the following: On one leg, you would treat SP 3 and SP 9; on the other leg, ST 36 and ST 43. One arm would be HT 8 and HT 3, while the other arm would be LI 3 and LI 11. This combination of points is made by using the image of the hand on the face (the whole torso, one full limb). I am also using the image of the full face on the full limb.

If you were choosing Master Tung points, your choice could be one leg 66.10 and 77.18. The other leg would be 77.08 and 66.05. One arm could be 33.12, San cha san, and 22.04. On the other arm, we could use 11.07 and 22.01-2. Using these points, I am using the image of the hand on the face (the whole torso on full limb), and I am using the image of the full face on the full limb.

The face image on the whole limb is not only effective, it is also less painful for the patient. I use this image almost any time I treat any face problem. This includes any sinus issue, face pain, eye issue, and teeth issue.

One thing I must say is that, in my opinion, acupuncture is not that effective for tinnitus. I usually defer to herbs for this condition. I have seen much better and more consistent results using ear acupuncture for tinnitus versus using body acupuncture points.

Yes, you can fix hearing problems from recent loud events or allergy-related dampness issues in the ear very easily. Age-related hearing loss and/or long-term nerve damage resulting in tinnitus is extremely difficult to treat with body points (regardless of the style).

Ear acupuncture and herbs are my preferred treatment for tinnitus. Have I treated tinnitus with Tung acupuncture? Of course, it works great. I just find that treating hearing problems is too "hit or miss" to say that I can be certain I am able to treat it effectively and consistently. I feel herbs and supplements are a much better choice.

Hand Acupuncture

Points 11.11-11.12 in Tung acupuncture treat spine-related problems. How can this be? They are on the dorsal side of the middle fingers. There is no acupuncture channel there, and the only channel even close to it is the PC. How can the PC treat the back? This is the theory of Kyoro hand acupuncture. I suggest anyone wanting more theory on hand acupuncture should study with Kyoro hand acupuncturists.

The middle finger is the torso. The ventral side of the body is the palmar surface of the hand. The dorsal side of the hand is the ventral side of the body. The second and fourth fingers are the arm. The fifth and first fingers are the legs. This is a great system with years of research to back it up. You can follow the images by watching your joints. Think about the second and fourth fingers as the arms. Each finger has three joints, and each arm has three joints (the wrist, elbow, and shoulder). The middle finger has three joints, and so does the back (C1, C7, L5).

The only issue I do not like about Kyoro hand acupuncture is the thumb. The thumb has two joints. The thumb in Kyoro acupuncture is the leg. The leg has three joints (the ankle, knee, and hip). It just does not line up for me. The fifth finger is the other leg in Kyoro therapy, and this does indeed have three joints. This lines up.

The homologous structure of the leg is not consistent with the thumb. It is for this reason I usually do Su Jok hand acupuncture. For me, it makes more sense. This is not to say that Su Jok is better than Kyoro hand acupuncture. This is not what I mean at all. For me, it just makes more sense to me, so I do Su Jok hand therapy.

I frequently use 11.11 and 11.12 for back pain. These are master points, but we can explain them very easily via Kyoro hand therapy.

Su Jok hand therapy, in my opinion, makes more sense. Su Jok hand therapy has the thumb as the torso, the second and fifth fingers as the arms, and the third and fourth fingers as the legs. This system for me fixes the issue of the thumb having only two joints versus the limb having three joints. The joints of the thumb line up with the joints of the back.

In Master Tung acupuncture, there is a point I use all the time for shoulder pain called Fan hou jue. It is on the base of the thumb at the proximal joint. This is a bit of a stretch, but the second joint of the thumb is C7/T1, and at the *same* level of C7/T1 is the shoulder. The Fan hou jue point is on the lateral side of that joint, where the shoulder is in Su Jok therapy. If we look at the human body, the shoulder is lateral to the C7/T1 joint juncture.

I strongly suggest further education in Su Jok and Kyoro hand acupuncture. If you do not want to take additional classes, you can simply memorize the Tung points on the hands. There are about thirty-eight points to remember, depending on how you group them.

The hand points are *extremely* effective, and I urge all practitioners not to forgo the finger points because you think they "might hurt." Yes, you do feel the needles more with finger points, but they are at times unmatched in their effectiveness. If you explain the benefits to your patients, they are usually willing to undergo a quick irritation of the skin.

Top Three Keys to Using Images and Mirrors Effectively

There are three things that are key to using images and mirrors effectively:

- Do not use the same image – layer your images
- One, two, or three needle approach
- Your patient does not know where the pain really is

Layer Your Images

The first key is do not use the same image. Use different images. An example might be headaches. We talked before about how the foot can be the head, the knee can be the head, the upper thigh could be the head (along with many other images).

You understand that there are many images, so do not use the same image. *If you choose to do more than the one body part, do not replicate it.* This has HUGE CLINICAL SIGNIFICANCE.

For instance, if you use 66.03 and 66.04 for headaches (located on the foot), and you want to use the other foot because the pain is bilateral, DO NOT USE the foot on the other leg. Choose a different image. Image the head at the knee, and use 77.18 or other points around the knee.

Then on the hand (again because you think there might be a reason for some additional points) do not use the hand or elbow. (You have already used this image on the legs.) You can choose a point on the arm that is in the upper jiao. Also, you would not choose the knee, hand, or mid arm. You would choose the fingers, such as the "tous," which are great for headaches and are located on the fingers. Every limb has a different image. This is a hypothetical patient, but the application is correct. You need to overlap your images. Layer your images by using different images. This makes a huge clinical difference in your patients.

Another example that makes a huge clinical difference is not to use just one image for one issue. *Layer it.* This means you can have three images for the eyes, or the lungs, or the heart, or whatever issue you are treating. This will ensure you do not miss the image or the relationship that is responsible for treating your condition.

Yes, it might be more than a few needles, and yes it may be too many needles. But if you layer your images, you will be more clinically effective, and your patients will come back. They will heal, and your practice will prosper. Once you are Dr. Jesus, you will need only 1-2-3-4 needles. Until then, overlap your images, layer your images, and be redundant in your images. It will change your practice instantly—I guarantee it.

An example of this is when I treat asthma. I use 1010.19-20 on the face. (It is one image and treats the lungs and kidneys.) I treat brachial ancestors on one arm, 44.10-11-12, which is great for asthma because it is right at the same level as the lungs and works wonderfully. On the other arm—Ling gu, Da bai, and San cha yi—these are different for treating the lungs, blood circulation, and warming the yang.

On one leg I treat 88.17-18-19, the Si ma points on the upper thigh. Then on the other leg, I treat 77.18-19-21. (With the lower leg image, SP treats LU, and the kidney roots the breath. In Tung acupuncture the SP, the earth, balances and treats the KD, the water.)

This is a much better treatment than treating the same Dao Ma on bilateral legs and arms. I am balancing multiple channels.

With these points, I have treated ST, GB, SP, LI, TW, and LU. I have used five different body parts for about twenty different images. This treatment is a great asthma treatment; it is much better than if I treat just bilateral Si ma points 88.17-18-19 on both legs. There is no doubt that will work as well, but by using multiple images, multiple channels, and more than six acupuncture points, you will do wonders for your patients and your clinic.

Using ONLY 1-2 or 3 Needle Approach

The second-biggest mistake I see distal practitioners make is the "1-2-3 needle" only needles. I am not referring to the 1-2-3 approach taught by my teacher, Dr. Tan, but the idea in Tung acupuncture that you can use ONLY 1-2-3 needles to fix any problem in any and all patients. Again, after you have seen 100,000 patients and inserted 1,000,000 needles, that idea is great. By then you *should* be able to use 1-4 needles and fix almost anybody or anything.

However, to get to 100,000 patients you will need to be successful in the eyes of your patients. That success is dependent on two things: your ability to run a business and getting fantastic results at least 80 percent of the time. I often see acupuncturists who are new to the Tung system using only 1-6 needles, using just one image, and using only one "Dao Ma" bilaterally for a condition. It does not work. The patient does not come back, and unfortunately, the acupuncturist will stop doing Tung acupuncture.

If you do not get results, you will not get the patients, you will not get the practice, you will not succeed in business, and you will fail. Where is this leading us? I want you to spread your image or mirror bigger than you think the problem is and use a few more needles.

Take knee pain, for example. If the pain is exactly at ST 36, there are many treatment options. We have discussed a few, such as 44.06, 11.09-11.13, and others. The best points, in my opinion, are around the elbow.

The best way to treat pain on the limbs is to use the same Chinese names. So foot yang ming is best treated by hand yang ming (the LI channel will fix the ST channel), and the MOST homologous structure is the elbow to the knee. This is the reason for choosing the elbow.

So if the pain is at ST 36 and you choose LI 11 to treat it, please add in LI 10 and LI 12. This will increase your chance of success by 75 percent. Needling above and below fixes this. You are, in essence, creating your own Dao Ma points.

It is interesting to note, is LI-12,11,10 not a "Dao Ma" just like Master Tung? That is three needles in a row for improved clinical effectiveness. Even Master Tung used two to three needles in a row to cure disease. If Master Tung did it, then I think it is a good idea.

System 1: Chinese Meridian Name Sharing, from Dr. Richard Tan

Shao Yin
Tai Yin
Jue Yin
Shao Yang
Tai Yang
Yang Ming

Meridian	Meridian
Du	Ren
Heart	Kidney
Lungs	Spleen
Pericardium	Liver
San Jiao	Gall Bladder
Small Intestine	Bladder
Stomach	Large Intestine

If the Du meridian is diseased, treat the Ren meridian. If the Ren meridian is diseased, treat the Du.

We have removed the Chinese names to make this simpler. If you just memorize this chart and know which meridians are paired, it is a lot simpler than remembering the Chinese names.

In my experience, the best channel relationship for limb pain is to use the name pairs, or System 1, as Dr. Tan teaches. This is the same system that Master Tung uses, called *Name Pairs*. They all work, all six to seven relationships, but by far, the System 1 name pairs is the most effective and reliable for limb pain.

>   Hand tai yin LU, balances foot tai yin SP
>   Hand shao yin HT, balances foot shao yin KD
>   Hand jue yin PC, balances foot jue yin LV
>   Hand yang ming LI, balances foot yang ming ST

Hand shao yang TW, balances foot shao yang GB
Hand tai yang SI, balances foot tai yang BL

All these channels can be reversed, so the SP balances the LU, the KD balances the heart, etc.

Your Patient Does Not Know Where the Pain Really Is

The second-most important idea is that your patient rarely really knows where the pain is. Yes, they tell where you where the issue is—the pain, the discomfort, the organ problem, the internal issue—but they know this only because nerve signals are being sent back to the brain.

They know only what area is receiving the most input into the brain. Yes, their kidneys hurt and they tell you that, but their liver could also hurt, or they could have digestive issues and they will not know this because the brain is focusing only on the worst problem at that moment, the kidney pain. By expanding your images, you will automatically address multiple issues.

If you still do not believe me, consider a patient with left-sided back pain who says, after you treat them, "Wow, my left side feels great, but now my right side hurts." You might reply, "The pain moved," but it actually *never moved*. It was always there. The proprioceptive and nociceptive nerves are not firing all that well. Because of the impaired firing of the nerves, you and I have a hard time telling where the pain is *exactly*.

You can close your eyes and burn your finger. You can tell exactly where you were burned. It is acute pain. The nerves—all the nerves—are firing. It is very easy to tell where the pain is, and what type of pain it is.

In chronic pain, the pain has been there for so long, (longer than three months) that the body starts to have a hard time telling exactly how the pain feels, and exactly where the pain is.

The reason they feel this way is that the left side was so painful that it overpowered the brain. The brain never told your patient the right side hurt as well because the left side was such a problem. Now that the left side is calmed down, guess what? The right side is still sending signals. Now, since the left side is quieter, the right side signal becomes louder.

This is much like two children crying. Where does your attention go first? If you have children, your attention goes to the loudest child first. Once that child has quieted down, you will then hear the second child crying. That second child was always crying, but you could not hear her because your son was crying so much louder.

Listen to and trust your patient. However, realize that your patient often does not really know where the pain is. They will not know the depth of their pain. They will have a hard time giving you the complete picture of their pain. They may or may not even know why they hurt. They may not know their asthma is complicated by their hypertension. They may not know their foot pain is really gout, and it is caused by failing kidneys.

They may not know they are depressed because they have a more urgent problem, such as diarrhea. In fact, 90 percent of your serotonin (your happy neurotransmitter) is made in your small intestine. As medical providers, it is our job to figure all of this out. However, remember, none of us are as smart as we think we are, and the body is still a great mystery on many levels. Every day medical research discovers something new about some disease it has taken for granted for the last fifty years.

By overlapping your images, using different images, and expanding your images, you take much of the guesswork out of distal acupuncture. These three ideas will improve your distal needling capabilities and increase your success by at least 75 percent immediately.

Master Tung wanted us to use few needles. The patients appreciate it as well. But as you learn, it is okay to use more needles. What is more important, to have a successful practice, happy patients, and wonderful results? Or to lose all of that because we failed as beginning distal acupuncturists, and we went out of business?

If we fail, then think of how many people will go without this amazing medicine. I do not think fifty needles is appropriate, but it is certainly medically appropriate to use five, ten, fifteen, or twenty needles on your patient as you learn and walk this path of Master Tung acupuncture. As I always say, "As few needles as possible, but as many as medically necessary."

Face and groin area

One image that I believe is very helpful is the one for the groin area. This is one of the most helpful images, even for local/TCM acupuncturists. The points at Ren 1 and Du 1, Ren 2-3-4, ST, SP, LV, KD are all in the groin area. There are distal images that I do not use in Tung acupuncture because they are on the mid upper thigh. The groin area is one that we should be careful when treating. Using an image or mirror is a perfect place to start.

There are many images for the lower groin area. The wrists, hands, and fingers all image the groin area. The feet and shoulders image the groin area. The other image I use quite often in the clinic is the face representing the groin area. We can theorize that the "top" of the head will treat the bottom of the torso, the groin. We can also theorize that the channels that end on the face, such as Ren 24 and Du 26, have their beginnings in the groin area, Ren 1 and Du 1. By treating the end of the channel, we can "balance" and/or treat the start of the channel.

The other image we have is the face itself. The eyes image the ovaries on women and the testicles on men, as well as the prostate. I know the distance of the testicles and prostate are different. From an image perspective it is the "shape" we are treating. The eyes are the shape of the ovaries, testicles, and prostate.

I frequently treat BPH (benign prostatic hyperplasia). BL 2 is one of my favorite points to treat the prostate. The nose is the penis and/or vagina/uterus. The lips represent the anus. The perineum is right at Du 26 (in between the anus and penis/vagina, and in between the mouth and nose).

Typically, if a person has hemorrhoids, you will see a small blue vein around his lips. I often bleed this to help with hemorrhoids. The points we would choose, either Tung points and/or TCM points, can further deduce what channels we are trying to balance.

The face in Tung acupuncture can be broken down by jiaos, upper, middle, and lower. These can be broken down further by twelve segments. There are many images and theories. The basic theory of the face is the channel relationships, with the face being an image of the groin. I do not use a lot of face points in my clinic, typically 30 percent or less. These points are remarkable nonetheless.

I have used face points to treat the kidneys and have helped patients actually get off kidney dialysis, which is not supposed to be possible. Again, I am not saying how great I am. Anyone can use Master Tung points. What I am saying is how amazing the Master Tung system is.

Some images and/or points that I use on a daily basis are BL 2 for any type of ovary, testicle, or prostate issue. The points 1010.09-10-11 are Tung points that are above the eyebrow. Although they are not indicated for ovary, testicle, or prostate issues, they are extremely effective for such conditions. The point 1010.22, Bi yi, is helpful to treat fatigue and back pain. I frequently use it for penis pain and vaginal issues.

It is interesting to note here that 1010.22, Bi yi, helps fatigue because of its relationship with the spleen. The spleen is responsible for dampness. Vaginal discharge is seen as too much dampness, or damp heat. This point is wonderful for it. The points 1010.19-20 are very famous points for asthma, breathing, back pain, and kidney issues in the Tung system. Again, although NOT indicated for anus pain or anus issues, these points are very effective.

For treatment, TCM point Ren 24, on the chin, is reflective of the lower groin. The Ren treats the Ren, and the Ren also treats the Du. Since both channels are in the groin area, they work great. We can use Du 25 on the tip of nose if a person has penis or vaginal issues. Du 26 can treat the perineum. The Du channel will treat/balance the Du channel itself, and it will treat and balance the Ren channel.

Treating both of these channels is very important when treating the groin area. I have also used Yin Tang and/or a point that is very similar, 1010.08, for treating nonspecific scrotum pain. When a man tells me his scrotum hurts and he doesn't know exactly where, I use Yin tang or 1010.08. These points, which are between the eyes, will treat between the testicles.

I think even if acupuncturists do not use a lot of distal points, they are helpful to treat the groin area, from both legal and professional standpoints.

Inguinal Crease

If you look at the crease in the shoulder, in the area of LU 2, that is the inguinal crease. Now if you work around the shoulder, i.e., posteriorly, you are moving posteriorly from the inguinal crease to the back. The lateral part of the shoulder will treat the lateral part of the hip. Now keep going posterior on the shoulder, and continue moving posterior around the back. Where the shoulder meets the scapula is where the PSIS (posterior, superior, iliac spine) is located.

The lateral edge of the scapula is the lateral edge of the sacrum. I can guarantee 100 percent that if you have pain on the attachment of the L5/S1 sacrum and you needle the superior lateral edge (you must hit the edge) of the scapula, you will knock out that pain, 99.9874 percent of the time. You should use two needles just to be safe, both about .5 cun from each other.

Full image or mirror on half a limb

Any time we image, there is always an image within an image, just as one of the most basic tenets we learn in Chinese medicine is that the macro is in the micro, or the micro is in the macro. We see the universe in the human, and the human in the universe. We are taught the yin within the yang, and the yang within the yin. Seeing another image is no different. It is the image within an image. This is a full torso image *now* on half a limb.

This whole torso image can be placed on either the leg or the arm, and it can also be reversed. It helps us make sense of many points and their indications. We can also put a whole limb on half a limb, such as a whole arm on half the leg.

The full limb is as follows, and remember it is reversed as well. The shoulder is the knee; the mid lower leg around SP 7 is the elbow. The ankle is the wrist with the toes as the fingers. This can also be reversed so that the elbow is the fingers, the mid leg at SP 7 is the elbow, and the ankle is the shoulder joint with the knuckle and toes being the top of the shoulder.

We can also place the entire leg on half the arm. The hip is the elbow, the knee is around TW 7, the ankle is the wrist joint, and the toes are the fingers. We can reverse this as well. The hip is now the wrist, the knee is around TW 7, and the elbow is the ankle. You can see already why the "Yao tongs" (extra TCM points), the "extraordinary back points" (literally translated), are so powerful. The hip in this image is right at the wrist. The Yao tongs are just distal to the wrist. If the hip is the wrist, then superior to the hip would mean we need to move distally to the wrist. The low back is superior to the hip, and the Yao tong points are just distal to the wrist.

This is why 33.08-09 are indicated for sciatica and leg pain. The lower arm can comprise the whole leg. The points 33.08 and 33.09 are 6.5 and 8 cun proximal from the wrist crease and .5 cun lateral from the TW channel. These points, being in the middle of the lower arm, represent the image of the whole lower leg.

Our image here of the hip is the elbow, and the ankle is the wrist. The length of the arm in between the elbow and wrist is the lower leg. Even if we reverse it, where the hip is the wrist and the elbow is the ankle, the lower arm distance between the two is still the lower leg. Do not most, if not all, sciatica patients have lower leg pain? These two points are needled on the lower arm to represent the lower leg.

We can continue to hypothesize and say, "Well, then I can also place the whole arm on half the upper leg, and I must be able to reverse it. This would then lead me to the fact that we can put the whole leg on the upper arm." And yes, again, we can reverse it. Clinically, we do not see this that much—the upper arms or upper legs used with the whole torso, or the whole arm/leg imaged on it. Clinically, you will typically see this image used on the distal part, i.e., elbows and knees distally.

For the longest time I could not understand why 88.25 or GB 31 was indicated for "elbow pain." How does the mid-thigh help the elbow? The full image of the arm on half the leg, the upper leg in this case, explains it. The hip is the shoulder, mid-thigh (GB 31, 88.25) is the elbow, and the knee is the wrist. We can reverse this. The knee is the shoulder, the mid-thigh is the elbow, and the hip is the wrist and fingers. This point finally made sense to me after viewing the full arm imaged on half the upper leg.

The whole leg can be placed on the upper arm. The shoulder is the hip, the mid upper arm is the knee, and the elbow is the ankle. This can be reversed again, so the elbow is the hip, the mid upper arm is the knee, and the shoulder is the hip.

The point 33.12, or heart gate, is located just distally to the elbow. If the elbow is the hip, then what would be just distal to the elbow? Just distal to the hip is the low back/coccyx. The point 33.12 is a very popular point for coccyx pain. Point 33.12 is just distal to the hip image of the whole leg being placed on half the upper arm.

It is not only full limbs that can be placed on half limbs; we can also do this with the torso. The entire torso can be placed on the upper arm. The head is the shoulder. The belly button is the mid upper arm. The elbow is the low back and groin area. This can also be reversed. The shoulder is the groin, the mid arm is the belly button, and the elbow is the head.

We explained earlier that LI 11 is good for dizziness because of the twelve segments, that any bone can be broken down into twelve segments, and that one segment was the head, LI 11. From this theory, we also see that LI 11 is the head area from the whole torso being placed on half the upper limb. We have already said how LI 11 could be the head via the twelve segments, as well as by placing the whole face on the limb. As always, there are many images within each image, and there is usually a way to understand an image.

We can also place the entire torso on just the lower arm. The head is the elbow, the mid lower arm is the belly button, and the wrist is the pubis symphysis with the fingers being the lower groin area. As always, we can reverse that image.

Clinically, I do not use the full torso on half the upper leg as much. It is much more common to use the full torso on half the lower leg. The theory says they both work—full torso on upper limb, and full torso on lower limb—but clinically you will find that the most success will come from the full torso placed on the lower limb.

This full torso image also applies to the legs. The complete torso can be placed on half the leg. The knee is the head, the mid leg is the belly button, and the groin is the ankle with the toes being the genitals. Again, we can reverse these images. We can also place the head at the hip, belly button/L2 at the mid-thigh, and the groin or lower back at knee.

This is one more reason why BL 40 is used empirically to treat low back pain. One of the many reasons it "works" is that the full torso is placed on half the upper leg. The head of the full torso is the foot/ankle, with the belly button being the mid lower leg and hip, and the low back being BL 40 area.

Shen guan, 77.18, which is very close to SP 9, is great for not only shoulder pain as we already showed, but also for headaches. With the entire torso being placed on just the lower leg, we see that the head is right where the knee is. Shen guan is 1.5 cun distal to SP 9. What is right below the head? It is the temple. Shen guan, 77.18, is known not just for headaches, but in particular headaches at the temple area.

The point 44.06 is known for many things. It is used for not only gynecological issues, but also nose problems. If we put the entire torso on the upper arm, the head is the shoulder. A few cun distally is 44.06, Jian zhong. If we come a few cun inferior on the face, what part do we bump into? You guessed it, the nose. Point 44.06 is an amazing point for stuffy nose, bloody nose, nose problems, and sinus issues. The whole torso of the body on just the upper arm offers one reason why this works.

Shen guan, 77.18., is famous for its ability to fix shoulder pain. We said earlier that the knee represents the elbow. How can the knee now be the shoulder? In this image, the *whole area* is place and "spread" or imaged on half the leg. The knee is the shoulder, the elbow is halfway down the leg, the wrist is the ankle joint, and the toes are the fingers.

Why is this a bit more difficult to see? I think the first reason is the number of "joints." We have only two joints now on the lower leg, the knee and the ankle, and yet on the arm we have three joints—the shoulder, elbow, and wrist. We have to imagine where the elbow is; we do not have a joint for it on the lower leg. We can also reverse this full limb image on half the leg. The fingers can be the knee, the elbow is on the mid lower leg, and the shoulder is the ankle joint.

We can already assume that, yes, imaging 77.18 or Shen guan for the fingers "does" work. However, we would ask if the knee looks like the fingers. In my opinion, it does not. I see a better image other places on the body. This does not mean you cannot use Shen guan/SP 9 for finger issues. I have done this in the clinic, and it "works" great!

We can also place the entire torso on half the lower/upper arm, or the whole torso on half the upper or lower leg.

The points 33.10-11-12—intestine gate, liver gate, and heart gate—are perfect examples of the whole torso on the lower arm. Point 33.12 is just distal to the elbow. The elbow is the head. Just below the head is the neck, and then the lungs and heart. Point 33.12 is just distal to SI 8, and thus is at the level of the heart; it is very effective for heart issues, hence the name, "heart gate."

If we continue distally down the arm, 6 cun up from the wrist joint on the SI channel is 33.11, liver gate. If we are imaging the entire torso on just half the arm, about halfway down the body is the liver, and halfway down the arm we find 33.11, liver gate, which is great for liver issues, hence the name. Just before we hit the wrist, the low back area, we find 33.10. Point 33.10 is only three cun proximal from the wrist crease on the SI channel.

If the wrist is the L5/S1 area, then what is at the level of L5/S1 pubis symphysis, the lower intestines? Point 33.10 is just proximal to the wrist crease. Without this full torso on half the limb, we would not be able to form an image perspective or be able to theorize as to why Master Tung used these points.

As we get to half and quarter, these images become more difficult for a few reasons. First, we are taking away the homologous relationships. We are also taking a larger limb or torso and putting it on a smaller area. This is just like ear acupuncture. The entire body is represented on the ear. If you are one, two, or three fen off (there are 10 fen in 1 cun), you will hit or treat a different body part. This holds true as we shrink things down to half or quarter images. We need to be more *specific* where we place the needles.

These full images on half the limb help explain why, classically, most acupuncture points were below the knees and elbows. The 5 antique points are below the elbows and knees. Why is this? Classical theory tells us why, but we now know that the most innervations, or the highest density of the nerves, are from the elbow and knees down.

The density of nerves continues to increase from the knees and elbows to become the densest in our halluces pollicus muscles (thumb) and fingers. This is why, clinically, most of your patients will wince when you needle jing wells, ying springs, or shu streams. The nerves are so dense in comparison to say the shoulder, back, or hip that the patient feels the intensity of the needle more.

In my opinion, this is why these one-half images at the knee/elbow have so many functions. These are joints where the nerve density is beginning to increase, and thus with the density of nerves, we have a bigger reaction in the mid cortex of the brain. You can also say we have a bigger "qi" sensation.

I do not confine myself to terms. You can choose any term or definition that "lights you up." As we find denser nerve bundles, we strike larger and larger areas of the mid cortex, and thus the reaction is increased. However, remember our guiding principal on "images" is what is the "best" image we can find? Which ones are the most consistent? It is important to understand them all, and it is even more important, clinically, to know which ones to use.

We want our patients to come back. We want and need our Western patients to feel a difference—today! Unfortunately, no matter how well I fix someone's kidney yang deficiency, if they still have back pain after my treatment, chances are they will not come back. Most of my patients *do care* about their overall health, and the kidney yang deficiency *is* important to them. However, they need to get to work tomorrow, and they need to be pain free today! They need to breathe today. They need to sleep today. Rain is wet and rocks are hard. That is how it is, usually, in the minds of our patients.

In my clinic, and I am sure in most acupuncture clinics, we get only a few treatments to help people. If we do not get results, our patients will leave. When I treat overseas, and it is a free treatment, I know my patients will come back. They will come five days a week, for three months. I can use any image because they all work. *They will all heal.*

I can use as few needles or as many as I want. It will work. They will not complain. They will allow me to make mistakes. Unfortunately, we do not have this luxury in a Western society, when patients are impatient to get fast relief.

Tissue Correspondence – Like for Like

"Homologous" is a term we used earlier to describe joints, bones, and muscles. Similar and like images are "homologous" in nature. As an example, the femur is homologous to the tibia. The second, third, and fourth fingers, for example, are just like the second, third, and fourth toes respectively. We said the lateral edge of the scapula was just like the lateral edge of the sacrum, and that the piriformis muscle was just like the teres major muscle.

There are other homologous relationships. This is the image of "like for like." There is a saying in Tung acupuncture that to treat bone, you needle bone. To treat muscles, you needle muscles. To treat tendons, you needle tendons. To treat the skin, you needle the skin (superficially). To improve circulation, you needle a vessel.

Though there is not an image of the body on the arm or the face on the leg, this is nonetheless an "image" of something. There is even research that shows that when we tap the periosteum of the bone, it increases bone growth by increasing osteoblast production. (Osteoblasts are responsible for bone growth.)

In the clinic, I have seen needles perfectly placed in the correct points and at the correct depth, but the needle does not yield fantastic results. This is usually because the tissue needled is not the correct tissue for the disease. An example is needling 77.01-2-3, which are for neck problems, in particular neck pain on the cervical bones. If you needle these points but DO NOT touch the posterior side of the tibia bone, your results will be only about 50 percent. It is the correct needle, and it is the correct point, yet we did not needle the correct tissue correspondence, in this case bone for bone.

A great example is a modified SI 4 point I was taught years ago. The needle goes from the HT 7 area up through the HT channel to the yang side of the arm. The needle passes just distally to the head of the pisiform and basically comes out at the SI channel. This is one of the best points I have ever seen for pain in the sacral joint area. Why is this? What does it image? What tissues am I treating?

The distal head of the pisiform is the image of the L5/S1 joint, and the tendon that it passes under at the wrist juncture is just like all the gummy tendon areas of the sacrum. It is quite an amazing point, but it works only if you slide it from the HT channel up into the SI channel. It is not an easy needle to thread through the bones.

The HT and SI channels treat the GB, BL, and KD channels. These three channels all run through the back. It is a great image of the low back. The wrist images the low back, and the tissue correspondence is perfect. The needle passes through a tendon, touches a bone, and goes through muscles. All three of these tissues are implicated in back pain.

Other great examples of this are LU 5, LU 5.5, and LU 6. The lower arm images the low back. The low back image is the T10-12, L1-2-3-4-5 area. The LU balances the BL, a very important channel in treating the low back. But what is so special about these points? The flexor and extensor carpi radialis are the big plump muscles that go down the LU channel.

These points are great for back pain. But what kind of back pain? Pain in the spine (bone) at the T10-12, L1-5? No. They are wonderful for back pain in the muscles at the level of T10-12, L1-5, which is around the quadatrus lumborum, lattissumus dorsi, thoracolumbar fascia; it will even, to a lesser extent, get the erectors and multifidus and the like.

However, these points are amazing for the meaty muscle pain in the low back. Because it is a great homologous representation of "like for like," the muscles are mostly the same. This is even better illustrated when you needle LU 5, LU 5.5, and LU 6 with HT 3, HT 3.5, and HT 4.75. Now I am treating both the HT and LU. The HT and LU will treat the KD, BL, and GB. We are picking up the three main channels in the low back.

The ulna also has good muscles on it. The image is correct, the channel is correct, and the TISSUE is correct. These points, although not Tung points, are some of the best points for T10-12, L1-5 muscular back pain. They will treat other problems as well, such as tendon, nerve, and bone at the T10-12, L1-5 on the BL, KD, GB channel. In theory, it should. But this whole book is about taking any needle from a decent needle to an amazing, therapeutically effective, 100 percent healing needle. Applying this step does that.

This same theory is applied to vessel or circulation problems. When treating circulation issues, we need to treat a point that has a "vessel" around it. We need to look no further than the brachial, radial pulse found on the upper arm. There are numerous places on the body where you can palpate a pulse, and it is interesting to note that we find acupuncture points at locations where the pulse is taken in Western medicine.

The brachial pulse is found in the upper arm. The Master Tung points 44.10-11-12, the three brachial ancestors, are great for overall circulation. The femur has the femoral pulse, a very large artery. Tung points 88.01-2-3 on the ST channel are indicated for all sorts of heart, circulation, and blood-pressure issues.

The liver channel is located on the medial side of the femur, next to the femoral artery. Points 88.12-13-14 are Master Tung points that are indicated for all types of blood deficiency and blood stagnation issues. The popliteal fossa at BL 40 is another area where Western medicine will palpate the pulse. Master Tung used this same location for systemic stagnation or systemic blood issues.

Yet another theory is applicable here. The tai yang has the most blood in it, so treating the tai yang vessel will move more blood. The posterior tibial artery is next to ST 36, or Master Tung points 77.08-09-10—11. These points in the Master Tung system are used for the heart and the lungs. They are most importantly used for blood circulation.

Having healthy blood flow through the heart and lungs is extremely important for the overall health of both of these organ systems. The more blood flow that goes through these organs, and through the channels, the better.

These points are also indicated for heart problems. Again, how do we fix a vessel? We must pick the right channel to treat it. We must pick the right *image* to image it, and we must pick the right *tissue* to treat it. Point 77.08 or ST 36 is both of these. The ST channel treats the ST. The ST channel runs through the heart, and the ST balances the PC.

The PC in Chinese medicine is responsible for the pumping action of the heart, whereas the heart channel is responsible for the emotional aspect of the heart, joy. The image is correct. If we put the whole torso on half the leg, the heart is right about at ST 36. In TCM, the master of the vessels is LU 9, which is right where we take the radial pulse. Interesting, is it not?

The last popular point is 66.04, Hou zhou. It is indicated for heart issues and circulation. Let us look at our theory. It is on the LV channel, so we balance the PC (in charge of the actual function of the heart). It balances the ST somewhat; it is jue yin, treating yang ming (that theory is a bit thin, but it works).

Usually, it would be the LV fixing the LI, but one can argue any jue yin will fix any yang ming. Its image is correct. It is in the upper jiao, and the heart is in the upper jiao, via the three jiaos for any bone. In this instance we would have reversed the three jiaos. Does the tissue match up? Yes! The dorsalis pedis is just under this point. It is amazing to see all our theories match up; that is what makes these points very effective.

The Si Ma points, 88.17-18-19, are very popular, and they are among the top ten most used points in the Master Tung system. They are indicated for many things, such as allergies, sinus issues, rib pain, and tinnitus. This leads us to our next theory, the theory on skin or dermatology issues. There are many reasons why these points can work for dermatology issues. One reason these points can be used for treating the skin is that when they are inserted very superficially, they affect only the superficial skin layer.

We needle the skin to treat the skin. If we needle deeply, we will activate the other indications because the nerve node that talks to the mid cortex in our brain is deeper than the skin level. I have also noticed in the clinic that when I needle deeply or moderately, I do not active the dermatological effects. When I need superficially, at the skin level, I see better clinical outcomes with the "skin." These points also work because of the five Zang fu lines, and this particular position on the leg is called the "lu" line, but that is another theory for a future book. Suffice it to say, when treating "skin" conditions, we need to treat superficially at the skin level.

The last relationship of "like for like" is the tendon. If we want to fix a tendon, we must needle a tendon. My favorite example of this is the ulnar tendon to treat the Achilles tendon. The Achilles tendon is sometimes "tricky" for us because there is no TCM channel located on the Achilles tendon. We have the KD channel on one side and the BL channel on the other side. There is no channel *on* the Achilles tendon per say.

So if we stick with our TCM theory, how can we treat the Achilles? Do we just needle the KD or BL and hope for the best? The Master Tung theory of like for like is perfect for this. Where is there a like tendon? Where would you find a tendon that is similar to the tibia and fibula tendons?

The radius and ulna are just like the tibia and fibula, and the ulnar tendon is just like the Achilles tendon. The tendon on the ulna is in between the HT and SI, just as the Achilles is between the KD and BL. The HT balances the KD, and SI balances the BL. The image is perfect, same structure for same structure. The tendon is like for like, just like the Achilles. If you needle *into* the tendon between the HT and SI, you will fix the tendon problem in the Achilles.

If your Achilles problem is mid lower leg, then needle the mid lower arm into the ulna tendon. If your Achilles pain is at the base of the Achilles, then needle the ulna tendon at the base of the ulna. If you just needle the HT channel and *come close* to the ulna tendon, or you needle just the SI channel and come *close to* the ulna tendon, then you will get only about 50 percent reduction in pain.

Understanding this "image," this "like for like," will help us understand why so many points have indications that may not make sense at first glance. This theory not only helps us understand many indications, but also takes our needling to a new level by making a good needle into a great needle. By taking a great needle into the perfect needle, that changes everything for the patient.

Tissue Correspondence Charts

This is just a small list of homologous tissue, muscles, and bone correspondences. There are more, but this will give you the most common ones.

Achilles tendon	Neck tendon/muscle
Anterior deltoid	Anterior groin muscles
Arm biceps	Biceps femoris
Artery at biceps 44.10-11-12	All treat the heart, all the vessels in the heart, and the lungs, overall circulation
Artery at femur	Aorta, arteries of the heart
Back of the arm	Is *not* the back of the leg
Back of the arm, triple warmer meridian	Side of the leg, gall bladder

C7/T1 joint	L5/S1 joint and vice versa
GB 34 joint	Joint on the ulna where it meets the humerus, not TW 10. Follow the joints.
Gluteal aponeurosis	Lateral deltoid
Gluteus	Posterior deltoid
Gluteus medial muscle	Lateral deltoid
Head of pisiform bone	Heel bone
Humerus	Femur
Iliac crest	Ridge on the scapula that is between the supraspinatus and infraspinatus
Interosseous membrane, between the stomach and gall bladder	Tendons and muscles between tibia and fibula
IT band	Triple warmer muscles on the back of the upper arm
LU 5/LI 11 joint	ST 36 proximal joint
Median nerve	No perfect image, the best image we have is the liver meridian. It is on a bone, but it still works well. This is the best image, even though it is not homologous.
Muscles on arm	Muscles on leg
Occiput GB 20, occiput BL 10	GB 40 joint, BL 60 in joint, modified
Piriformis	Teres major
Radius	Tibia
Scapulas pushed toward the spine	Sacrum, lateral scapula is lateral sacrum
ST 41, deep space near this point	Hip and shoulder joint (deep pain). ST 41 is most homologous to LI 5 wrist pain
Shoulder bursa	Hip bursa
Shoulder, clavicle	Pelvic girdle and hip
Side of the arm, large intestine meridian	Front of the leg, stomach meridian
Spleen 4	Head of the distal joint on thumb bone
Toes	Fingers
Ulna	Fibula
Ulnar tendon	Achilles tendon

Vascular	Artery at foot 66.03-4, 44.10-11-12, 88.01-2-3 etc.
Vastus lateralis	Large intestine channel from LI 15 to LI 12, the deeper arm muscles
Wrist bones	Ankle bones

Image and Mirror, Homologous Structure

One must understand the terminology first of what an image and a mirror are before we can explain this theory. A mirror is something you have *two* of on your body, or at least one other thing that is alike. So *mirroring* is like comparing your feet to your hands. You have five fingers and five toes. Each toe and finger has the same number of joints. The bones are a "homologous structure," a "mirror." Dr. Tan taught me this terminology, and I continue to use it as well.

Some examples of "mirrors" are as follows: Your tibia and fibula are mirrors of your radius and ulna. Your femur is just like your humerus. Your ankle joint is just like your wrist joint. Your shoulder joints are just like your hip joints. All of these things are mirrors. Every part of your body has something that looks just like it. This holds true as well for muscles and tendons.

The ulna tendon is like the Achilles tendon. The muscle on the ST channel of the leg is just like the muscle on the LI channel on the arm. The muscles of the back match up. The piriformis is just like the teres major. The posterior deltoid is a mirror to the gluteus. The bursa of the shoulder is a mirror to the bursa of the hip.

An *image* is something that *represents* the thing you are trying to treat. For example, you have only one head. Nowhere else on your body do you have another body part that is like your head. So how can we treat this? There is no *mirror*. However, there is an *image*. An image would be the representation of your hand being your head. Using this image, the fingertips would be the top of your head. The distal knuckles would be your forehead.

The PC 8, HT 8 area of the palm of your hand would be your eyes/teeth. The palm of your hand would be your chin. Your wrist joint would be the C7/T1 joint. As we work our way down the arm, we are working our way down the spine.

As we reach the elbow, it is an image for the belly button and/or the T12/L1 area. There are many points around these areas that make sense. LI 11 is great for digestion. The image of the intestines is at the belly button.

As we move down the spine, we move up the arm. The bicep/tricep area represents the L2-5 zone. As we approach the shoulder joint, we are imaging the L5/S1 joint and the pelvis. The coccyx images the acromion, or the top of the shoulder.

This is an *image*, which is something that we are trying to make be like something we do not have. These two terms are paramount to understanding what we are talking about when it comes to mirrors and images.

How would we image your heart? You have only one heart. We need to find a location on the body—typically a limb, but it could be anywhere—where we say, "This spot represents/images the heart."

You have only one set of teeth. We have to find a place on the body that treats it. This would be an image. A very popular place is typically around the elbows or knees, for example.

From a mirror perspective, let us forget about channel relationships for a moment. What is similar to the mirror of your first finger, distal joint, at the ulnar side? Your first toe, distal joint, at the ulnar side, would represent this area.

How would you mirror the area that is four inches proximal to the knee joint, but using the arm, not the leg? The exact mirror would be four inches proximal from the elbow joint down the radius. A mirror image of your mid forearm, 1 cun lateral to TW 4, would be on mid lower leg 1 cun lateral to about GB 39. So, mirrors are relatively straightforward.

How would we mirror a muscle? We need to find a muscle that acts and functions in a similar way and has the same structure. My favorite example is the teres minor for the piriformis. Both of these muscles are in between the ball-and-socket joints of the hip and shoulder. The muscles have the same function, and if you were to needle the teres major, you can almost guarantee that area will treat pain in the piriformis.

Another example could be the biceps of the arm and the bicep femoris of the leg. They both have "two" heads of the muscle. They both function the same; they both look the same. They are, in fact, mirror muscles of each other.

The muscles, attachments, tendons, and ligaments are all the same in the toes and fingers. These joints look alike, and they act alike. They have the same attachments of muscles and ligaments. They have the same number of joints. The movements are the same. All the muscles, tendons, and ligaments are mirror images of each other in the toes and fingers.

The next step in using mirror images is figuring out which channel to use once you have found the spot, the mirror. There are seven channel relationships. There are six channel relationships that are widely taught, and there is even a seventh relationship. Essentially, you will use only about four channels to treat any issue. However, we do need to be aware that there are more channel relationships than just the four I discuss here. We will discuss this later.

All seven channel relationships will work, but what I want to know, and what I am sure all the readers want to know, is what is the best channel, or the most reliable channel you can choose? You will most likely use *mirrors* when you are treating *limb* issues. When you treat torso issues, you most likely will be doing *images*. However, there is another kind of mirror that I would like to explore.

This *mirror* is a homologous tissue. Homologous means "corresponding or similar in position or structure or function or characteristics; especially derived from an organism of the same species." We have already discussed how the radius and ulna serve and look just like the tibia and fibula. We have said the fingers look and act like the toes. The shoulder joint is just like the hip joint, which is a ball-and-socket joint. Many things on the human body are similar in appearance. The question is, are there other homologous relationships that we can "mirror"? The answer is yes.

I would suggest the "point zero" of the body is in the middle of the torso. If you look at the back or the front of a human body, there is a "center point." We are looking at *just* the torso. In your mind, cut away the arms, legs, and head. We are left with the *torso*. There is a center point on the torso. That center point is the xiphoid process, or Ren 15 or T9 area.

That center point has *no* homologous structure. It is the exact *middle*. It is a starting point. This can be a little different depending on whose "torso" we are viewing, but usually the xiphoid process is at the same level as T9, and it is at the exact center of the torso, or the starting point.

The back is a complete mirror, or better said, a homologous structure. Put both hands on T9. As you move 2-3-4-5-6-7 cun inferiorly, move your hand 2-3-4-5-6-7 superiorly. All these structures are mirrors for each other. You can treat pain at T1/C7 and pain at L5/S1. They are the same. If you move your hand from the sacrum laterally over the gluteus, it is the same image as taking your hand and moving it from the scapula across the posterior deltoid to the shoulder. The scapula is still a mirror, but somewhat of an image.

If you take both scapulas and "push" them together, they become a mirror of the sacrum. The lateral edge of the scapula is the lateral edge of the sacrum. The teres minor and major muscles are the piriformis muscles of the low back. These are homologous structures.

Locally, you can needle the piriformis and affect the teres major and minor. You can needle gluteal muscles and affect the lateral and posterior deltoid muscles. You can needle into the sacral bone and fix pain in the scapula. You can needle the S2 joint space and affect C5-6 joints.

This all becomes important because there are hundreds, even thousands of images to choose from or "make up." The question always is, "Which ones work the best?" It does not matter what image you use. *The most consistent and reliable results come from the images that are homologous in nature.* We will discuss throughout the book what images produce the most consistent, reliable results.

To elaborate, let us look at the possible images for treating low back pain. I will not name them all, but you will quickly see how many images we can discuss.

The shoulder can represent the low back. For example, Pian jian, a Tung point, and/or TW 14, SI 10, and LI 15 all represent and treat low back pain. These points are most consistent with joint pain in the low back because we are needling into joint spaces. Usually this will get the joint space of the low back, L5/S1 area, PSIS (Posterior, superior, iliac spine), etc.

We can also "reverse" our shoulder image. We now have the shoulder as the head. As we move our way down the arm, the elbow is the belly button, and the wrist/fingers are now the low back. We can needle the TCM Yao Tongs for low back pain. Ling gu, 22.05, 22.06-7-8-9, and SI 4, are all for low back pain.

We can choose the ankle to represent the low back. We could needle around the ankle using either Tung or TCM points. Now, the question we should be asking is how do we avoid inserting thirty needles into someone? Which points will give us a great result with the least amount of patient discomfort? We also want to know which points are the most reliable.

We can needle the fingers to treat the back, 11.11-12. We can needle the face to treat the back, 1010.22 and 1010.19-20. We can needle the head to treat the back, 1010.25. We could needle, I would say, any bone or structure and affect the back. Which points produce the best effect for our patients? Of all those bones, images, or ideas, which would be the best? That depends on so many conditions, but in a "static" situation, the best image is the homologous one with the appropriate channels used to treat the disease.

Out of all of those points and images, which image looks the most like the hip joint? The ankle and wrist joints are similar to the low back. We can see the resemblance. However, do not the shoulder, arm, and scapula look much more like the hip and low back? The shoulder has a ball-and-socket joint, just like the hip has a ball-and-socket joint. The scapula looks just like the sacrum, and the upper arm looks just like the upper leg. These are by far my favorite points, day in and day out, for low back pain. The image is amazing, and the homologous structure is perfect.

Can we think of a perfect structure to treat the shoulder? In my experience, the best way to treat the shoulder is the hip. Again, the *mirror* is perfect and so is the homologous structure. In America though, it is not always correct or convenient to treat the hip. Where else do you see a mirror or an image for a shoulder joint? We can *reverse* the image. So, the ankle is the wrist, the knee is the elbow, and the hip is the shoulder. Then we can also say the ankle is the shoulder, the knee is the elbow, and the hip is the wrist.

Now, is this the best way to treat the shoulder? No, it is not. *We are not using the best homologous structure.* However, in America this is the best we can do. There are other images as well of the shoulder, but I wanted to show clearly that there are times when picking the perfect mirror, or homologous structure, is not always applicable or appropriate.

We will continue to explore additional images, mirrors, and homologous relationships. These terms are important to know and to be able to distinguish. A *mirror* is different from an *image*. When you have multiple mirrors or images to choose from, a few ideas will guide your choices. Certainly, personal clinical experience will be one way to choose. Patient comfort, how they are dressed or undressed, and how they are positioned if lying on the table are others. Lastly, the mirror or image that is *most homologous* will be the best choice when choosing what mirror image to use.

You will continually hear about System 1 limb pain. This means that when we have pain on the limbs, we choose the same name pairs to treat each other. For example, LU treats SP, HT treats KD, PC treats LV, LI treats ST, TW treats GB, and SI treats BL. These relationships go back and forth, so the LU treats the SP, and the SP treats the LU, and so forth.

There are seven different channel relationships. They all work, but by *far* the "name pairs" work the best for limb pain. We have to ask "why" this is. Is it luck? Is that just how it is? I think it is because when we use the "name pairs," the channels, for example LU and SP, are completely homologous. The resemblance is in the bones and the muscles. It is quite amazing. Look at LI and ST. The muscles are completely homologous.

Does the LI treat the LU? Yes, it does. It does it very well. However, look at the structure of the muscles, arteries, and veins. They are different from the structure on the LU channel. Does the BL treat the LU? Yes, it does. It does it very well. However, look at the structure of the muscles, arteries, veins, bones, and bursas. It is *different* from the LU.

Now look at the SP. It is anatomically perfect! It is perfectly homologous, and this is why I think "name pairs" for pain on the limbs are therapeutically effective. This theory has been tested on tens of thousands of patients, and by many other acupuncturists. The appropriate channel for the LU could be the LI, BL, or the SP. The SP will *always* produce stronger and more reliable results with pain on the limbs.

For the torso, or internal problems, we will choose a different relationship. This is applicable only to pain on the limbs. I struggled for years to understand why "name pairs" were always better. It is only by understanding the homologous relationships that we are able to choose the best image and/or mirror.

Quarter Image

This is where it gets a bit maddening. I do not use or see this image used as much as the other images, but it is worthwhile to explain it.

The quarter image is where you place the whole arm on one quarter of the leg (typically the lower leg). Or, you can place the whole leg on a quarter image of the arm (again, the lower arm). I do not know why, but typically when theorizing quarter images, we do not associate it with the upper leg or upper arm. Also on the quarter image, there are not a lot of points and/or theory to reversing the quarter image, even though you can.

This is where things can break down. It is much like Newtonian mathematics. Newton's laws work great in the "normal" world, but as we get super big, Newton's laws break down, and we have to use Einstein's theory of relativity. As we get super small on a quantum scale, we need to forget Newton and Einstein and shift our thinking into quantum physics. This quarter image is much the same.

Some of our theories will break down as we get too "small." This also becomes problematic, much like taking a copy of a copy. Have you ever noticed what happens if you copy something, then make a copy of the copy, and then make a copy of the copy of the copy? Little imperfections that were not seen on the original start to show up on the copy of the copy of the copy.

If you copy the copy long enough, you are left with an image that will not even resemble the original. This is much like taking images down to a quarter, an eighth, or a sixteenth; it gets so small that little imperfections that were never noticed before become huge issues for our treatments.

The quarter image is not used as much for a few reasons. One reason is that you are making your image so small it becomes difficult to determine exactly what is what. Secondly, there are already a few theories that deal with "small spaces," such as the three jiaos or twelve segments theories.

Four points that come to mind and are used a lot are PC 6 (and/or PC 6 and 5) and 77.20 (1 cun proximal to SP 6), 77.09 or around St 38, and 77.24-5. PC 6 and the Dao Ma of PC 6 and 5 are used to treat knee pain. The entire leg is put on a quarter of the arm. If the hip is the mid arm, then the midway point is between mid arm and the wrist. Using PC 6 and/or PC 6 and 5 for knee pain is very effective. In my experience, there are great theories or reasons at work here, but from an image standpoint, no other "image" makes sense other than a quarter image.

It was understanding this quarter image that enabled me to see the "why," or at least part of the why. Again, I would argue in Tung acupuncture they do not reverse the quarter image. However, to explain theory, we will do that. You can also apply the quarter to the upper arm, though not many points fall within this category.

The point 77.20 is indicated for shoulder pain and four-limbs pain, but mostly for shoulder pain. I was also curious as to how a point that is one cun proximal to SP 6 could help with shoulder pain. The quarter image is at work here. The entire arm can be placed on the mid to lower leg. The point 77.20 is right about mid to lower mid leg; thus via the quarter image, this will help the shoulder joint.

One can even argue that this might even be an eighth of the image, but now we are splitting hairs. Every image has an image within it, and this point works for many reasons, but from an image perspective it shows us that a quarter image is applicable.

The point 77.09, or around the area of ST 38, is a famous point as well for shoulder pain. This nicely matches up with the whole arm being on a quarter of the lower leg. The yang ming, 77.09 located in the area of ST 38, is a same side yang point treating yang shoulder pain. According to our theory, *yang points treat only the opposite side*. The theory also says that yin points can treat the same side, and/or opposite side, but yang points treat only the opposite side.

In this case, ST 38 or 77.09, treats *only* the same side. Nobody has a theory as to why. I have posed this question many times to the upper ranks of the Tung community, and the answer I always get is, "Well, it just is same side." It is interesting to note, and you can try this on patients with bilateral shoulder pain, if you insert 77.09, or the TCM ST 38 area, you will find that almost 100 percent of the time that only the *same* side of the shoulder is fixed. Not the opposite shoulder, like you would expect.

The points 77.24 and 77.25 are on the lateral side of the leg about where ST 38 or 77.09 is. Again, this same relationship plays out. The points 77.24 and 77.25 are known for their effectiveness for digestion and throat issues. They are used for shoulder pain. This full arm being placed on a quarter of the leg, much like ST 38, shows us that this works.

From a theoretical perspective, there are quarter images on the upper leg, but we do not see them that much. What we do not see is the quarter image reversed. Although it is interesting to discuss theory, in a clinical setting it is a moot point. Our objective is to find the most reliable points to treat our patients. I have yet to see a point where the quarter or eighth image is used and reversed. These images get so small, a copy of a copy, that reversing them, I am assuming, would be just too many copies of a copy, and it would not work that well.

I think these images explain many points, but a better point they explain is the image of an image, a reversed image, again half-imaged, flipped over, and turned around images. They do work via theory, and sometimes we can "spin a yarn" to make any point make theoretical sense, but be careful with splicing down and flipping images too much. We can lose sight of the original and be left with only a highly fragmented copy of a copy that does not resemble our original piece of artwork.

Three Jiaos

In Master Tung acupuncture, any bone can be broken down into three parts. These three parts represent in general terms an "upper," a "middle," and a "lower" jiao. The most famous of these "bones" that is broken down into three parts is the second metacarpal bone of the hand.

Ling gu, 22.05, is at the base of the second metacarpal joint, and 22.04, Da bai, is at LI 3, though many Tung practitioners would argue for 1,000 years where exactly 22.04 is. Just for sake of argument, let us say that Da bai, 22.04 is LI 3. I have also included a TCM point, LI 4, He gu, to use as an example.

Ling gu helps lower back pain, gynecological issues, and groin issues. LI 4 is known in TCM for being the "master of the face point." LI 4 is also great for most types of stress and/or digestion issues. The TCM point LI 3 and/or Da bai, depending on your teacher, is known mostly for helping with headaches. It is also a "helper" for Ling gu. There are over sixty indications for Ling gu alone. I want to focus on the concept of the three jiaos, not every indication of Ling gu and Dai bai.

Applying "general" imaging, you can see why Ling gu, the lower jiao, is effective for what I have mentioned. Being in the middle of the hand, LI 4 represents the middle of the body and thus helps with stress (the liver, in the middle of the body, i.e., the four gates, the small intestine where 90 percent of the serotonin is made), and it improves digestion. The SI/LI, ST/SP, pancreas, and GB are all in the "middle of the body." Then LI 3/Da bai is great for "head issues" being in the upper jiao.

You can also reverse this image, so in essence, Ling gu would or could be the upper jiao. TCM point LI 4 is still the middle jiao. Now, LI 3, Da bai, is the lower jiao. In theory, this is correct. One will find, though, that the more we reverse, chop, splice, copy, and change, the less effective your point selection will be. LI 3 or Da bai is *not* very effective for low back pain. Ling gu is very effective for headaches. In my clinic, I will frequently use Ling gu for headaches, and I am applying the reverse image of the upper, middle, and lower jiao concept.

There are numerous examples. If we look, we can see this idea repeated over and over. Great new research proves GB 34 is wonderful for stress. GB 34 is on the tibia bone. GB 34 is at the upper jiao of that bone. We know LI 11 is great for blood-pressure reduction. LI 11 is located on the radius bone. If we break down the radius into three sections, the upper middle jiao, then LI 11, is either at the low end of the lower jiao or the upper end of the upper jiao.

LI 11 is great for headache reduction, especially if it is caused by hypertension. It also treats dizziness caused by hypertension. It still works great for any headache or dizziness, but typically, it works better if the headache or dizziness is caused by a heart issue.

There is a point combination in Tung acupuncture that is extremely effective for many odd, random, and autoimmune diseases, as well as any type of stagnation issue. These points are called 77.27 or the three lateral passes. It is a set of three points evenly distributed on the GB channel along the fibula.

I suspect that the reason this three-point combo is so effective is that we are treating the upper, middle, and lower jiaos at the same time. Whether we reverse it or not, these three points cover the entire body. The Three Emperors is another very popular Dao Ma in Tung acupuncture. Tung points 77.18-19-21 are on the spleen channel and are distributed in three sections. They affect the upper, middle, and lower jiaos.

One can look at the indications of these points and now have a deeper understanding of why it is that 77.18, or Shen guan, is used for headaches. It is in the upper jiao. There are a multitude of other theories as to why it works for headaches, but with our three-jiao theory it makes complete sense.

SP 6 is relatively close to 77.18, which is located at the Three Leg crossing point, which is one of the most frequently used points in TCM for lower gynecological issues. SP 6 and 77.21 are in the lower jiao. The spleen is used in TCM for insomnia and stress, and upper neck and back pain. If we reverse the jiao, SP 6, 77.21, is now the upper jiao. And is not SP used in TCM for insomnia? Stress? It is also used for upper neck/back pain. SP 7 or 77.19 is in the middle jiao, and 77.18 is in the lower jiao.

This concept of the three jiaos is paramount to understanding the treatment of the body as a whole being, and to how we provide a holistic treatment. Rarely in complicated cases is one needle going to be enough. Rarely is low back pain just back pain. They may have inflammation of the liver, a bit of constipation, some blood stagnation, qi stagnation, inflammation of the spleen or kidney, degeneration of the spine, inflammation of a disc, tight muscles or tendons, and even a genetic deformity.

Low back pain, although easy to treat, is usually much more complicated than our patients or we can determine. This is where the idea of the three jiaos comes into play. We know Ling gu in the lower jiao will alleviate low back pain, but back pain does not exist in a vacuum. There are other issues at play, ones our patients and we often do not know.

We certainly know of health care issues. We are also aware that we do not know all the health problems at any given time. Therein lies the complexity of our human understanding of the beautiful inner workings of the body. Just as we use only 10 percent of our brain, we may really understand only 10–25 percent of the total health care issue at any one point, whether we are Eastern or Western trained. The three jiaos take your guesswork out of it. You give the power back to the body. You let the body regulate the three jiaos, and with harmony, comes health.

How would we apply this? Typically our patients need much more than just a "general" treatment and/or a "general idea" of what treatments to do. We need to be very specific in our treatments points. If I do not know exactly what to do, and/or if my patient has many complex issues, I will defer to the strength and knowledge of the body. I will focus on the theory of the three jiaos.

When I apply the theory of the upper, middle, and lower jiao, the treatment is very effective. Never think that we know more than the body does. If the disease is too complex, it may be too difficult to be a "perfect 1-2-3 points" to fix your patient. However, a more general approach is needed if this person has a disease in all jiaos, or all body parts, and I do not know where to start.

I may typically employ 22.04-.05 and LI 4 on one hand. Then on one leg I will use the three lateral passes 77.27. I allow the patients to rest for two to five minutes, and then I can recheck. How are they feeling? Is the pain reduced? Do they feel an improvement? The results are nonetheless remarkable, and it takes a lot of the guesswork out for the practitioner. This is not my preferred method of treating. However, this is the theory of a holistic nature of treating the entire person.

Some people may ask, "Well, if I am treating the middle jiao, what *exact* part am I treating?" Using *only* the theory of the three jiaos, we do not know. Remember, for each point we pick, you might have ten to fifteen theories as to why it works.

You will see points that are extremely effective and that usually have more "theories" to explain them than the points that have only one to two theories explaining them. I would like to emphasize that I do not mean they are less effective; they are just less reliable. They will be used for more specific issues caused by specific problems.

For example, Ling gu is such a great point for low back pain. It is on the large intestine channel, which balances the kidney channel. The kidney channel is in the low back. Ling gu is in the lower jiao, using the theory of the three jiaos. Ling gu is a twelve segment. The twelfth segment is the lower extremities. The reaction area of Ling gu is the lungs but also the ischia bones (sacral bones).

Ling gu is in the joint space of the first and second metacarpal. It is a homologous image of the joints in the low back. Ling gu is on the yang ming channel, the channel with the most qi and blood. Typically, pain is qi and blood stagnation. These are just a few of the theories that we can discuss about ling gu. You will find in your clinical practice that the more theories a point has, the more effective it is.

An example of this is PC 6 and LV 3 for knee pain. PC 6 is our treatment point and LV 3 is your guide point. PC 6 is a quarter image, tendon for tendon, and PC balances ST. There are only three theories as to why this works. It does treat wonderfully, but it will only treat knee pain on the ST channel when the cause is patellar tendonitis. It is very specific, whereas other needles or other points have multiple theories for their treatment of knee pain and are more widely used.

Can we think of another bone that can be broken down into three parts? Any bone can be, but how about the femur? Points 88.12-13-14 are called the three upper yellows. As per the name yellow/jaundice? I am sure you can already guess what they treat in the "middle jiao." Yes, these points are typically most often indicated for liver problems. They are located in the middle of the thigh on the liver channel. They are in the middle jiao. Could they also treat GB, ST, SP, and the intestines? I would argue yes.

Another point that confuses most Tung practitioners as to why it is so great is GB 31, or 88.25 (they are the same location). Point 88.25 is one of the most important points in Tung acupuncture. It is most known for "pain anywhere in the body." How can this be? GB 31 or 88.25 is in the "middle." It is at the middle point of the femur on the GB channel. How could one point in the middle jiao help pain anywhere?

We know using other theories why it works, but can we explain it using just our three-jiao theory? Can we explain why putting a needle in the middle jiao will help pain? Inflammation comes from the spleen. (According to Western medicine, the IgA, IgE, IgG, and IgM are all inflammatories that circulate in our body and cause us pain and inflammation.)

Perhaps this is why so many "powerful" pain medications suppress the immune system. Examples of this are prednisone, Enbrel, and methotrexate. Again, we are treating the middle jiao. The spleen is in the middle jiao. By generally bringing back balance to the middle jiao, we reduce the systemic inflammatories that are circulating in our bloodstream, thus reducing pain.

If we can fix the middle jiao and/or the spleen, we will have less pain, less inflammation, and better digestion. Remember that 90 percent of our serotonin comes from the small intestines. Serotonin makes us happy. Good digestion means more smiles and less pain. Now, does seeing GB 31, 88.25 (top point for pain and stress in Tung system) or LI 4 as being great for stress and digestion make more sense?

The three-jiaos idea is a broad concept to understand. How can one understand the trees if we do not take a step and see the whole forest. It is a mistake to think we can look at one tree and grasp the entirety of the forest. Acupuncture points are at times like this, a "tree." The three jiaos of Master Tung allow us to still see the "tree," but also to be able to step back and treat the whole forest. If the whole forest is healthy, then of course the trees are vibrant. But even with the healthiest 1-2-3-4 trees, your forest can still be diseased.

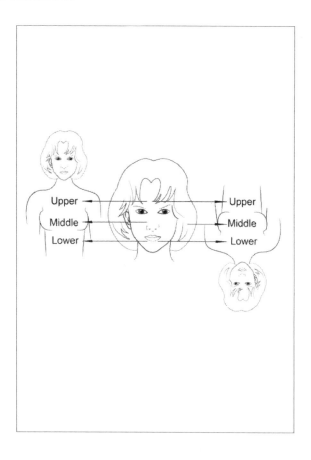

Theory

In mathematics, there is a paradox of movement and infinity. It states that an arrow in flight will never hit the ground. How can this be? Theory and mathematics say that there are any number of ways it can be divided. Therefore, ten can be divided by two to make five. Five can be divided by 2.5. And so on to infinity. We can reach our goal because we can always divide that last distance—any distance, no matter how small—by two.

If the distance from the arrow, in mid-flight, is ten feet, and the ground is zero feet, then in theory we should always be able to divide that infinite space by two and still have some distance to move. The arrow should never reach the ground. But it does. Reality says it does, and we can watch the arrow go through the sky, and yes indeed, it hits the ground. But theory says that is impossible! There is an infinite number of numbers; mathematics has proven that. We have proven that the arrow does in fact hit the ground. We both have proven we are right. But we are both not right. The arrow does in fact hit the ground, no matter what we do.

Theory is wonderful and I enjoy it, but be careful because theory is not reality. We use theory to explain the "why," but it does not always matter "why." In our clinic, sometimes the outcome trumps any theory we might try to use.

I have studied with one of the most prominent pulse takers in the world. He basically changed the way you take pulses, much like Master Tung certainly revolutionized the acupuncture world. I asked him one day how he came up with his pulse diagnosis. It is from the classics, no doubt, rooted in tradition, but he took it to a whole new level. It was the "whole new level" that I was trying to understand.

He told me that in the hospital where he worked, he would just spend all day in the kidney ward, or the heart ward, or the cancer ward. He would feel the pulses of those patients whose diagnoses were already established. Then he would work backwards. He would feel the pulse and say, "Okay, this is a kidney-dialysis patient, and this is the pulse they are presenting with."

This is much like the theory of the "arrow." Our theory says the arrow will not hit the ground, but if we are to completely understand or "jump-start" our thinking, we have to put theory down for a second and *just observe*. What is happening? What is

71

the outcome? Wow, the arrow hits the ground. This does not really match the theory. We will need a new theory to explain this. If we stay stuck in our mode of "theorizing" everything, we will get in the way of ourselves.

Consider the ancients and the five elements. What came first, the five elements or the world? The world was obviously made or created, or whatever your idea of creation is. Humans came later, much later. The earlier Daoist doctors looked around and tried to make sense of the planet. They created the "five elements" to explain their reality. Again, we should ask NOT about the five elements, but we should be asking why NOT four elements? Why were there not six? Why were there five?

Once the five elements were developed, they worked backwards to make the five elements fit the world. They did not theorize the five elements, and then the world came made to fit into the elements. Some of the most amazing theories were first NOT a theory. They observed, watched, realized a result, and then worked backwards to make it fit.

I would think Master Tung was much the same. The depth of Master Tung's theories is amazing. However, be careful. I think it was not his theory that made his points amazing. He found amazing points either on purpose or by accident then worked backwards to figure out what theory would rationalize his points.

Master Tung was a master of the fourteen TCM channels. These were the same TCM channels you learn in TCM school. Most people think Master Tung used only "Master Tung special points." He did both. Master Tung used their "special and unique" family points, and he used the fourteen TCM channel points. This is why so many Tung points either overlap a TCM point (same location, but Tung usually had a different indication 33.16/LU 5, 88.25/GB 31) or Tung points are very close to TCM points.

So the question is, did theory guide him to these special points, or did he by chance place a needle in a just a little different location, and then watched with amazement at the results. I think it was both. Take for example Men jin, 66.05. (There are hundreds of examples.) Men jin is very close to ST 43. It has some of the same indications, and it has some different indications, from TCM ST 43. So, did theory guide him to this point? Or was this point mis-needled one day? It was supposed to be an ST 43, and by accident, he or someone else placed it where Men jin, 66.05, is now located.

The location is basically ST 43, but it is more proximal. The point is right at the juncture of the second and third metatarsal bones. It is only about .3-.5 cun difference between ST 43 and Men jin, but Men jin is a much more powerful point. So here was this needle, which they thought was in ST 43, but the outcome they observed in the clinic was different. Why was this? They went back and, I am assuming here, noticed this point was producing new outcomes. They examined the point again, and sure enough, they saw it was in a different location. They rationalized what they saw in the clinic and worked backwards to apply the theory to this new discovery.

Take for example 77.08 and ST 36. They are both in the same location, but the Master Tung point is closer to the tibia than ST 36. Most people have said, "Well, this makes sense. In the "old" days, their needles were much thicker and rudimentary, so ST 36 was moved from the bone so as not to injure the bone and tibial artery. This makes sense, but why did Master Tung not move his needle farther away? Their family certainly had rudimentary and "old" needles as well.

Again, I think this point was needled by accident, and I bet, closer to the bone one day. They saw different indications than expected and started asking questions. Why is this needle producing new or different results? Then they applied the theory to these new indications and worked backwards.

The whole point of this explanation is to draw attention to the fact that it was not the theory that produced the discovery of these points. These points were treated intentionally because they wanted to see what would happen. Or they were needled by chance, and then the theory was applied. If we get obsessed by having only theory guide us, we will never get out of the way of ourselves to discover new points and/or let the arrow hit the ground.

Here is an interesting side note on both 66.05, Men jin, and 77.08: They are both very close to the TCM points ST 43 and ST 36. What is the difference? They are both closer to the juncture space, 66.05, and closer to the bone, 77.08. It is interesting because these points are so much more powerful than their previous locations. Is this theory? Does theory tell us that if we move our needle a few fen up or down we will have a better outcome? No, it does not.

However, what is happening is that there is much denser webbing of nerves, muscle attachments, ligaments, and tendon attachments as we get closer to the metatarsal juncture. This higher density of tissues will cause a stronger reaction in the body, and thus bigger and wider therapeutic applications. It really is quite amazing.

Some people say, "Well, who cares about imaging or mirrors? There are so many images and mirrors. Any point we pick must be a mirror or image of something, so it must work. Just stick a needle anywhere, and we are bound to get some image of an image and it will work. Or we can reverse, half this, quarter that, flip this, and change that. I can image any image anywhere for anything." You can, but it does not work that well.

I always urge against this thinking. Even if you put the needle in the wrong place, it has some effect, but it will not do much. It is true, yes, as Western medicine says, "Who cares where you do acupuncture? The results are always the same." This is not really accurate. It is true that regardless of where we needle someone, there is a systemic increase of blood flow, endorphins, nutrients, and healing properties circulated *everywhere*. And yes, no matter what, some healing takes place.

This is not a "put down" to acupuncture; it shows only how amazing needling the body really is. We can needle anywhere and cause some change. How miraculous! No matter what you do, you will cause some healing! Wow! In Western medicine, if they do the wrong thing, they kill people.

I remember volunteering in a retirement home. My youngest patient was seventy-six and my oldest was 104. It was fun. I was a new practitioner, and I did not have a lot of experience. I remember saying, thinking, and seeing that it did not matter where I put a needle. These patients were so old, so sick, and had so many complications that even one needle in the thumb seemed to help at least a little.

The question and quest for any practitioner is not learning new things, but how do I take what I already know and make it better? How do I take a needle that gives me a 50 percent improvement in health or a 50 percent reduction in pain and make it a needle that gives me a 75–100 percent improvement?

We learn acupuncture to figure out how to take a decent clinical outcome to an amazing healing experience. We should not be happy with just 50 percent with Tung acupuncture, or any style of acupuncture for that matter. Our goal should be at least an 80 percent success rate. As we master this medicine, I would personally hope to see a 90–95 percent success rate. I think right in now in my clinic, I have an 85 percent success rate. This includes both complex and simple cases.

This brings us back to images. Yes, there is always an image of an image. Yes, we can make up so many images that in "theory" any image should give us a good clinical outcome, but this is not true.

We need to look no further than the point Ling gu. This point is indicated for back pain, among many other things. According to theory, Hou zhu, 66.04, is the exact same point on the foot that is just like Ling gu. These are the same points on the same type of digits. We can apply all the same theories to each of these points, and yet 66.04 does not relieve back pain the way Ling gu does. Why? Our theory says *it should*.

We can look at 77.09, which is ST 38. It is an amazing point for shoulder pain (more on this later). All our theory says to needle the opposite side. Yet for this point, we do same side needling. Why? According to the theory of channel relationships, the I ching, Ba guas, and all our theories, it should be the opposite side, yet it is the same side.

Take for example the area of LI 8. According to our theory, if so above, so below. It is the micro in the macro, and the macro in the micro. The yin within yang, and the yang within the yin. Any bone can be broken down into anything. So why does this point, in the area of LI 8, not work like 77.09 or ST 38? They are the same exact location.

Why do all points not do the same thing? Our theory might confirm this, or at least we could spin a theory as to why it may or may not work. Why do they not work? They just do not. The theory, though beautiful and helpful, is still just that, a theory. Theory will help guide us, help us understand, help explain our natural environment. Just like our medical ancestors chose the five elements to help them make sense of the outside environment, our theory helps us explain the complexity of the Tung system.

Make no mistake, the theory is *not* why these points "work." These points work because they work. I would think these points helped therapeutically, and then most people worked backwards trying to find a theory as to why they worked.

The theory does not make it so; it is so because it works in real life on patients. The arrow hits the ground because it is so; it just is. We have to think back to where our theory fails us in mathematics, just as with Tung points. The points work, practiced over 2,000 years by Master Tung himself on over 400,000 patients and family lineage since 200 BC, passed down from father to son. The theory helps our mind make sense of a healing capability that we don't yet fully comprehend.

The other thing you can do is just memorize everything. But memorization is boring, difficult, and static. There is nothing in Chinese medicine that is static. The medicine is continually evolving, changing, and progressing much like our diseases. Take Wu-hu 1-2-3-4-5 points in Master Tung. Originally, it was said Master Tung used this point only for big toe pain.

The Wu hu points are on the lateral aspect of the thumb. It makes sense; the thumb treats the big toes. And what part of the big toe? Master Tung said the inner aspect of the big toe, just as the needles are on the LU channel of the thumb. (LU balances SP.) But now in the year 2000+, we have adapted these Wu hu points, 1-2-3-4-5 to have *many* more applications. Wu hu 1 treats finger pain, Wu hu 2 treats wrist pain, Wu hu 3 is just a helper for the other points, Wu hu 4 treats foot pain, and Wu hu 5 treats heel pain.

In just thirty to forty years, the indications and applications of the points have shifted. That is quite amazing. There are now also other acupuncturists who have found and adapted the big toe to be five new points on the big toes. The big toe is the 5 Wu hus of the big toe. We will have to use these points for the next 100 years to see if they work just like the thumb Wu hu points. But the point is that things change. Thirty years in medicine is much like the blink of an eye. That is a very short time for things to change. Nothing is static; we are all changing.

Another illustration of this concept is that theory says the yin channels balance or treat not only the yin/yang channels opposite, but also the same side yin channels. We also know that the yin channels balance or treat themselves, and they have their paired yin channels that they treat. If we pick three yin channels—for example KD, LV, and SP—our theory says we are treating the opposite side and same side HT, PC,

LU, and opposite side TW, LI, SI. So the opposite arm is completely covered. If I chose the right KD, LV SP? Then I have already balanced ALL SIX CHANNELS on the opposite arm.

With the same side arm, the same also holds true. The yin balances the yin, and the yin also balances the yang. So the same arm is completely covered. Now look at the legs. KD will treat BL, LV will treat GB, and SP will treat ST. We cannot really treat KD, LV, and SP on the opposite leg, but our theory also says you can treat the pain or issue with the EXACT spot on the opposite limb. So if we treat KD, LV, and SP issues on the one leg, we can take the KD, SP, and LV on the opposite to treat it.

Okay, now we have the opposite leg completely covered via theory, so now for the same leg. KD will treat KD, LV will treat LV, and SP will treat SP. The only thing KD, LV, and SP will not do is treat the yang channels on the same limb. But that is okay. Our treatment points are on the right, and we are treating left arm pain. We already said we have 100 percent of the left arm balanced.

We have not discussed what the KD will fix. It will fix the KD, HT, LI, TW, and BL. The LV will fix the LV, LI, PC, and GB. The SP will fix the SP, ST, TW, and LU. The only channels we cannot fix are the Ren and Du. This is okay because the Ren and Du do not run down the arms. So no matter what, we have all six channels balanced and treated in the left arm with our right leg three yin channels.

Now we have to pick an image that treats all images. We can image the whole left arm on the right leg. We can also image the entire left arm on half the right leg. We can also take the whole left arm and put it on a quarter of the leg. That quarter image can also be reversed. So if I needle all three yin channels on the right leg, on a quarter image, about two to three needles per channel spacing out the needles, I have treated that whole image.

So we have all the channels covered. We have an image up and down reversed that covers the whole arm. So in theory, no matter what issue comes up on the left arm, I have it covered! I have tried this numerous times. But the arrow hits the ground, and doing acupuncture this way does not work even though theory says it should.

Another illustration of this concept is that the theory says the yin channels balance or treat not only the yang channels opposite, but also the same side yang channels. We also know that the yin channels balance or treat themselves and also have their paired yin channels that they treat. If we pick three yin channels—for example KD, LV, and SP—our theory says we are treating opposite side HT, PC, and LU and opposite side TW, LI, and SI. So the opposite arm is completely covered.

There will be conditions that are not treated this way. The theory starts to break down. Use theory as a guide, as a choice, but it is in the clinic, with our patients, that we prove if it works or if it does not. I enjoy theory; it is fun. It gives us ways to remember things. This whole book is about imaging and mirroring. Remember that it is the imaging and mirroring that are used to *explain* these fantastic points. The points work with or without the theory. They just work.

Inguinal Crease

Pain, and in particular back pain, is the most commonly treated condition in acupuncture. Many acupuncturists struggle to treat back pain. The back can be very difficult to treat. I have suffered with intense low back pain. The main reason I became an acupuncturist, rather than a Western MD, was that alternative medicine was able to cure my low back. Western medicine just gave me pain medication and had me scheduled for surgery. It was my back pain, and the Ling gu inserted into my hand, that transformed my focus to Master Tung acupuncture. Never before had I felt acupuncture results like that. It was, as I say a lot, an incredibly miraculous healing needle.

There are many images and points that treat "back pain." We can image the wrist, the extra points in TCM, the Yao tongs, the fingers, and Master Tung points 11.11-12. We can image the elbow for the low back 33.12 or 44.02-03. We can image the upper arm or mid lower arm; these both represent the mid lower back. We can image the same joints on the legs.

We can image the ankle points BL 65-62-60 (a Tung Dao Ma by Dr. Maher), the knee, BL 40, an empirical point in TCM for back pain, and/or the upper thigh, 88.25. We can image the face for back pain, 1010.22, 1010.19-20. There are so many images from which we can choose. The one image I have not mentioned yet is my favorite: the shoulder joint and scapula.

I like this image the best for two reasons. The first reason is that it is much less painful to needle the shoulder than the wrist, ankle, toes, or fingers. I think this is an important consideration in your treatment plan. Certainly, this does not guide my treatment plans, but we do need to consider patient comfort if we want to run a successful practice. (Most Western patients are not as comfortable with acupuncture as they did not grow up with it.) The second and *main* reason I always defer to this image is the "structure." It is a *perfect homologous structure.*

The humerus is just like the femur. The shoulder crease treats the inguinal crease. The anterior shoulder treats the anterior femur. The bursa of the shoulder treats the bursa of the hip. The lateral deltoid treats the lateral hip/femur. The posterior deltoid treats the posterior hip and/or the gluteal muscles. The posterior aspect of the humerus, where it connects to the scapula and the shoulder girdle (almost where SI 10 is) is the lateral edge of the L5/S1 joint. If we needle into that joint space in the posterior shoulder, we are treating the L5/S1 joint. Where the shoulder meets the scapula is where the PSIS (posterior, superior, iliac spine) is located.

When we start to go posteriorly down the lateral edge of the scapula, we are going down the lateral edge of the sacrum. The teres major is the piriformis. Go back to our theory of "tissue for tissue" of the Master Tung system. It makes sense that the thick muscle of the teres major is just like, looks like, and has the functions of the piriformis.

In addition, if a patient has pain on the sacrum and we needle the scapula and *miss* the edge of the scapula, it will not be that therapeutic of a needle. If we needle the lateral edge of the scapula and tap the bone? Then the needle will 100 percent treat the bone, ligaments, and all the bony connections of the lateral sacrum. Many times you can treat the lateral edge of the scapula to fix piriformis pain because the root of the pain is the origination of the posterior muscles on the sacrum and the attachments.

Using this image, how would we treat sciatica? The first question we need to ask is where is the sciatica? Is it on the posterior, medial, or lateral side of the leg? All these questions would guide our choice of channels to treat. The best image would be the posterior shoulder joint and the superior lateral edge of the scapula.

True "sciatica" comes from the S2 nerve root. All other radiating pain down the leg is really called "radiculopathy." The posterior shoulder joint would treat the joint of L5/S1, and the superior lateral edge of the scapula would treat the S1-2 area. These few needles may be enough to stop the pain and the radiation. I will usually also include needles that run inferior down the SI channel aspect of the arm. This is assuming the sciatica ran down the *posterior* leg of the patient.

I will use two to five needles running down the arm. If the patient can *specifically* tell me where the radiation is, I can target that area. If she says it just goes down her leg, I will use two to three needles, starting on the superior posterior, SI aspect of the arm. I put each needle 2-3 cun distally down the channel. You normally do not need to put needles all the way down the channel, even if the patient has pain all the way down the leg.

It is common to confuse the correct image with the arm being the leg. The lateral aspect of the arm is the LI channel, but the superior aspect of the leg is the ST channel. The posterior arm is the TW; the posterior aspect of the leg is the bladder.

The posterior medial aspect of the arm is the SI channel, whereas on the leg, there really is no yang channel at this same image. What happens is if the patient has posterior back pain, you might think you could just treat the posterior arm. *This will not work.*

The TW posterior arm will not fix the posterior leg on the BL. *To fix the BL we need to treat the SI.* (There are five different channels to treat the BL, and TW is not one of them.) The patient might say she feels pain on the lateral aspect of her leg. If we go to the lateral aspect of the arm, it is the LI. The *LI will not fix the GB.*

The lateral aspect of the leg, the GB, matches up with the posterior aspect of the arm, the TW. Often the patient will say, "I feel it wrap around and go down the front of my leg." The anterior part of the arm is the LU channel. The LU channel will not fix the ST.

The anterior part of the ST is treated by the lateral aspect of the arm, the LI. With all these yang channels of the leg, there five different channels to treat them. Unfortunately, the LU does not fix the ST, the LI will not fix the GB, and the TW will not fix the BL.

Most other body parts line up correctly, but when it comes to the arms and legs, due to Chinese anatomy, we have to be careful to first choose the correct image, and second to choose the correct channel to treat it/balance it.

Scalp Image – How to Avoid Du 1 Treatments

There are many "scalp images" that can be used with great success. In regards to Tung acupuncture, Master Tung placed C1 at Du 24. As we move posterior along the Du channel along the hairline, we are progressively walking down the spine.

Master Tung point 1010.07 is just posterior to the hairline and helps with headaches, stress, and head issues. You might say it is a local point—it is a head point used for head conditions. I agree it might be. It is what we call a "close distal point." In my opinion, the image here, the C1, the atlas, the top of the spine is the reason it treats head issues.

Would we needle this point if the patient had a headache at this *exact* point? I think not. We have over 740 points from which to choose. Another point would make more sense therapeutically. I frequently use 1010.07 for upper neck, and C1 for spine pain. It is interesting to note here that out of all the seven channel relationships from which we can choose, only the Du channel has two relationships that balance, as does the Ren channel.

The Du channel will treat itself, and it will treat the Ren channel. The Ren channel will treat the Ren channel and the Du channel. There are no other channels that will treat the Ren or the Du. Therefore, if we want to treat the Du channel at the C1 area, 1010.07 is an excellent choice via channel relationships and image.

In many cases, treating the Du channel is your only choice to treat the Du Channel. This is why "imaging" the spine on the head is so important. The Du is treating the Du, and the image of Du 24 is correct with C1. We can insert this needle either superficially or perpendicularly. I prefer a *superficial* insertion because I get more length on the Du channel.

Points 1010.01-5-6 are basically the Du 20-21-19 respectively. They have spinal indications and stress, anxiety, and depression indications. From the overlay of the spine image, we are treating "about" T10-12, L1-2,-3-4. DU 20 or 1010.01 is typically the landmark of "L2."

Du 20 is an interesting point from the three-jiaos and multiple-images perspective. Du 20 will treat pain under the chin. The top of the head will treat the bottom of the head. Again? What part of the chin? It would treat only Ren or Du imbalances. Du 20 will also treat Du 1 issues or Ren 1 issues. The top of the Du treats the bottom of the Du. The top of the Du will treat Ren 1. Du 20 will also treat heel pain. The top of the head will treat the bottom of the foot. (More about this later.)

As we continue further in a posterior direction, the next "landmark" we reach is the EOP, the external occipital protuberance. This is Master Tung point 1010.25. It is a two-point unit; both points are inserted superficially *toward* the EOP. They both treat Du pain in the low back area, in particular the *sacrum*.

I will never forget my first one-needle treatment. A woman in India had had an epidural seven years ago. The scar of the epidural was *right on the spine* and right at the sacrum area. Theory would suggest that long-term pain, even though on the Du channel, would have migrated to the kidney vessel; kidney is bone. If we need to fix bone pain, then we should be thinking bone or kidney.

In this case though, I hypothesized that treating the Du with the Master Tung point 1010.25 would fix this, as long as we "tapped the bone." (More on this later: to fix the bone problem, we must needle the bone.) I used one needle, and her pain instantly disappeared. My patient and I were both equally surprised. I was out of school for only five days, and here I was in India treating 100 people a day. I was there for three and a half months, and just before I left, this woman came back and told us that after that one treatment she was pain free, 100 percent, and her pain had not returned since. That is the power of acupuncture.

The spine overlaid on the image of the head is very powerful indeed. At times it may seem confusing. We know where C1 is, at Du 24. We know where L2 is, at Du 20, and we know where the sacrum is, the EOP. Where is C3? Just a bit posterior to Du 24.

Where is T7? I would suggest it is one cun anterior to Du 20. Where is T11? It is .5 cun superior to the EOP. There is always a bit of variation in these spots. That is why I suggest you needle *superficially*, so your needles cover more surface area.

I would suggest in the beginning that you insert two to three needles. If the pain is located between meridians, ask your patient if the pain is gone. If you chose correctly, the pain will be gone, or at least 80 percent in one inhalation. I always ask patients to breathe once, then check how they feel. I do not ask how they feel. I ask *where the pain is now*.

The biggest mistake practitioners make is to not be aware that the spine pain is located on more than just the Du meridian. You may fix the Du, but remember the BL and KD are also involved. It is also possible the patient might have an internal problem. The pain could be located on the anterior side of their body, but it is referring to the posterior spine.

As always, theory would say that we can "reverse" this spine image. I and other practitioners have found that in this case, it does not work to "reverse" the image. Remember, theory is a guide; it helps us, it teaches, but clinical application *proves* our theory. Until we prove it, theory is just that; it is theory.

I do not know why, but reversing this image does not work. Sure, we can argue it does work. I am sure some patients have responded to a "reverse" image of the spine on the head. The question is always, which image is most consistent? Which is therapeutically most effective? It is the image of Du 24 representing C1, Du 20 being L2, and the EOP being the sacrum.

Belly Face

One image we have not covered yet is the stomach area representing the face. An acupuncturist friend of mine had a patient a long time ago who had migraines for over ten years, but only at the area of yin tang. Other than migraine headaches, she had no other health problems.

Being a TCM (local) practitioner, she treated the liver and gall bladder meridians, with little effect. In most cases, there is a gall bladder or liver meridian pathology with migraine headaches. When the normal migraine treatments did not work, she decided to unblock the area on her forehead using points to open that meridian.

Her treatment principle was to do multiple points around Ren 12, on the Ren meridian, to open the Ren. Of course, she did not realize at the time that she had forgotten where the Du began and the Ren ended, as you tend to forget those things when you have been out of school for a while. She inadvertently treated the Du meridian by needling the Ren meridian. After a few treatments, the patient was completely well.

After learning about the Master Tung Dao Ma theory, she realized she made her own Dao Ma. She had not heard of Dr. Tan at that time, so she had no idea that she was balancing the Du meridian via the Ren.

In TCM school, we learn that Tai yang belongs to the Du channel. We already said that the Du meridian can treat the Du and Ren. The Ren meridian can treat the Du. These are our only two channels to choose from, except for a few Dao Ma's in the Master Tung system that are related to the Du channel.

In this instance, she chose several points on the Ren meridian (Ren 12, 13, 14) to treat and balance the headache at yin tang. It worked immediately. The image she was using was the abdomen being broken down into an image of the face, just as Du 20 will treat a throat condition just under the throat.

The head is a complete unit. The top of the head, Du 20, treats the bottom and the underside of the chin. If we expand this image, now Du 20 can treat the next segment in the bottom, the anus, or Du 1 area.

If we continue this segmentation of the body, the "bottom" is the bottom of the foot. The Du meridian is indeed wonderful for heel pain. The top of the head treats the bottom of the foot. The face is no different. We can image the face on the abdomen. We have said before that the elbow, the knees, or the belly button are the "eyes." In this case, the points were just above the belly button, Ren 8, and she needled Ren 12, 13, 14, or in that area.

What is just above the eyes? Yin tang is just above the eyes. We can even see the reverse of this. In Master Tung acupuncture, 1010.10 and 101.10.11 are Si fu er and Si fu yi, which means "bowels second and fist point." They are right about the eyebrows. Their indications are acute abdominal distention, hangover, etc. The eyes are the belly button, knee, and elbow. So here, Master Tung points are using the imaging system, but in reverse.

To further delineate where the images line up, the forehead is the upper stomach, lower chest area. The area around Ren 17 is the image of the middle forehead. Up to Ren 22 would be the top of the head, and Ren 2-3-4 would be the chin area.

The eyes are again at the belly button, and just above or below the belly button is just above or below the eyes. This, of course, can be reversed. The forehead can be the Ren 4-5-6 area, with the top of the head being Ren 2-3-4. Ren 22 would be the bottom on the chin, and the area of Ren 17 would be mid chin to lower lip.

The other image that is important is the front for the back. It is not a half or a quarter image; it is that the front will fix the back, and the back will fix the front. In the clinic, because all my patients lie face up, I am doing more of the front to treat the back. This is how this theory is applied. The Ren and Du only balance each other. I often needle Ren 24 to treat neck pain. The point at the chin balances Du neck pain in the back.

If my patient has low back pain on the Du channel, I can needle the Ren channel at the corresponding level. So if Du 4 is painful? I would needle Ren 3-4-5 to treat and cover Du 4. Remember to always expand your image. If we are treating Du 4, we want to treat a little above and a little below to make sure we cover it.

This idea or theory would also work if the patient had pain on the GB, KD, or BL meridians of the back. You can pick the corresponding level on the stomach and needle that channel. That is the theory. However, in practice, I have found that when needling the front for the back, I can needle at the exact same level as the back pain and treat at the *exact* same spot as the pain.

So if the pain is around your quadratus lumborum on the left side, you would treat the left side on the belly and *exactly* where the painful point is in the back. If your needle "could" go all the way through the body, in theory, it would touch the point of your pain. Obviously, you do not needle from the front to the back, but to explain it, I think that makes sense.

Of course, if you treat many people lying face down, you could treat the dorsal part of the back for the ventral side. I think if we look at many of the "back shu points," this theory holds true. In Master Tung acupuncture we never needle the torso. We only bleed the torso. In Master Tung acupuncture the points on the back that are bled for a specific organ always "happen" to be right behind the organ they are treating.

I do not use this theory a lot; I rarely needle the torso. For those people who do, this is a wonderful theory and a clinically effective way to treat many conditions. There have been times when nothing else would work for a patient's back pain, and it is the 4-5-6 needles I place in the abdomen that resolve it. Follow your system, but do not be bound by your system. Walk the path, but also know when to step off the path.

Information on Case Studies and Letters

Do I heal every patient? No way! The case studies and letters presented in this book help to illustrate and highlight "mirroring and imaging." Do all my ideas work all the time? No. I have spent seven years treating about 65,000 patients in multiple countries with Tung acupuncture. I have failed, learned, and failed again, but I continue to try.

I am not saying this to boast, but if I can be successful in a small town of 12,000 people doing Tung acupuncture on all my patients, so can you. I am not special. I see 100 people a week with no contracts and no advertising. My patients show up or come back because of the clinical results. The results are not from me; they are from the Tung system that I use. I have no secrets and no golden needles. I do not have privileged information. I know of no "ancient Chinese secret." What I know is studying, trying things out, observing, and learning from our failures.

Anyone can do this with a little time and effort. I think the amazing thing is that I am a beginner and it still works. (I think everyone is a beginner until we treat a minimum of 100,000 people.) I do not know very much and it works. It works in my town where nobody likes, believes in, or wants to get acupuncture.

Do I change my mind all the time with points? Yes. At times, I can have ten patients with low back pain and use ten different theories and points on all ten patients. Acupuncture in a book or a case study is a very "static" thing. There is nothing further from reality when practicing in the clinic.

My mind is constantly weighing and cross-checking. Is this point worth it? What will this do? How is the patient? Is she stressed? Is she happy? Does she like acupuncture? Do I have her trust? How is my time? What is the length of the treatment? Is my diagnosis right? Am I guessing? What will happen tomorrow? Has this patient had acupuncture before? All these things come and go when treating a patient.

I also use herbs, supplements, a cold laser, cupping (rarely), and micro current for local point stimulation. (I do have some patients who just *need* to be stimulated locally. I do that with a micro current device.) In five years, will my point selection change? Of course it will. We are always learning, changing, and thinking, and yes, my point selection will change. This is why I always stress theory and understanding the nature of the points.

Really, in the end, there are no points. There is a human body in front of you, and with the correct stimulus and by utilizing many theories, we can effect a change. There are an infinite number of points and channels on the body.

This concept is similar to what I experienced when I used to compete in sports. You must learn the movement, the exercise, and the technique. Then you must forget it, if you want to perform at a top level. A top athlete does not *do* the movement. He/she *is* the movement.

You do not think to *do* this or that; you *are* this or that. This is what acupuncture eventually becomes for all of us. As you read my case studies and letters, realize they are for educational purposes, to illustrate how this system can be used.

By no means is this a manifesto on how to treat any particular patient. There are too many unknowns and details to either write and/or describe to any one person. We can learn the reality of this system only by experiencing it. This is only a theory about how it all works, until we use it ourselves and see the results.

Here is one of my favorite quotes:

> Far better is it to dare mighty things, to win glorious triumphs, even though checkered by failure ... than to rank with those poor spirits who neither enjoy nor suffer much, because they live in a gray twilight that knows not victory nor defeat.
>
> **Theodore Roosevelt**

Our books, letters, and case studies are a starting point. It is up to you to go out into the field of medicine, draw your lance, and strike out for new lands. Then you will know both failure and glorious victory.

CHAPTER 3

SECRETS TO SUCCESS

Master Tung, who was born in 1916, has a family system of acupuncture that has quickly become one of the most effective acupuncture styles in the last twenty years. Master Tung acupuncture includes more than 700 acupuncture points. Some of these points lie on, or are the same points that were mandated by the People's Republic of China. These 365 points, and hundreds of others, were "discovered" by the Tung family, thus making this style unique and effective.

Master Tung's belief was that "chronic illness" gave rise to Bi Zheng (rheumatism/pain/systemic chronic disease). Master Tung treated "chronic illnesses" not with just one needle here or there, but he organized his family points into groups of three needles in close proximity to each other along a meridian. This became known as the "Dao Ma" effect. Master Tung concluded that just one needle on a channel was not enough to clear or cure chronic or systemic illnesses (Dr. Maher Advanced Tung acupuncture).

Most of the common issues any acupuncturist will see in the West will be long-term issues, chronic in duration, and insidious in nature. The "Dao Ma" concept is perfectly adapted for these types of diseases. Over 60 percent of Master Tung points are organized in Dao Mas, thus showing us that this "concept" of obtaining "De qi" is very important.

We now know that the stronger the reflex is in the cerebral cortex that we get doing acupuncture, the greater effect it will have on the organism. Master Tung's main belief was, "The quicker we bring De qi, the quicker the results will be."

The Tung point numbering system is as follows:

		Number of points
1	Fingers	27
2	Palm and dorsal hand	11
3	Forearm	16
4	Upper arm	17
5	Plantar aspect of foot	6
6	Dorsal aspect of foot	6
7	Leg and calf	28
8	Thigh	32
9	Ear	8
10	Head	25

One point on the heart meridian, 22.10, which is the hand-release point, shows that the Tung acupuncture points predate the heart meridian. This point was passed down from father to son from the year 200 BC. There are also 200 or so points on the chest and back; these points are treated by bloodletting therapy.

There are many theories as to why Tung acupuncture works so well. I have tried to organize what I would suggest, in my personal experience of 65,000 treatments, that I use the most. I use all the theories, but the main focus in my teaching is to determine which one works best. Which theory is the most consistent? Which ones can I bet my practice on? The following information is what I stake my practice and patient satisfaction on.

Guiding and pulling

Always use the same channel, same side. Using the same side to treat pain is known as the guiding/pulling technique.

Overlap channels

It is always best to overlap the channels. If you have back pain on the bladder meridian, where the kidney and bladder are involved, do not treat the bladder channel bilaterally. Treat the bladder meridian on one side and the kidney meridian on the other.

If your patient has a headache on both sides, on the yang ming meridian, do not do LI 4 on both sides. Do LI 4 on one side and LU 10 on the other side. Treat ST 36 on one side and LV 3 on the other. *That makes a huge difference in your treatment outcome.* All of those channels balance the large intestine.

IMAGES

(There about 10,000 images. The following are the most commonly used.)

- Draw a line from the torso to the limb, and needle that area. Be careful, though. This theory does not work that well for areas that have joint problems, necks, backs, etc. I only use or like this "drawing a line" for internal issues.
- If you have mid back pain, draw a line to the arms. That line would hit the mid upper arm. Needle that area on the arm to fix the back. (Obviously, choose the correct channel in that particular area, and make sure your line is "hitting" the correct homologous structure.)
- Hand is head; elbow is mid abdomen; the shoulder is low back.
- Foot is head; knee is mid abdomen; the hip is back.
- Put the whole face on arm; put the whole face on leg. (Elbows and knees are eyes.)
- Arm is the leg; leg is the arm.

The Most Consistent and Reliable Images

The more distal you get, the more reliable your results. So fingers/hands to feet/toes are more reliable, and vice versa. It is interesting to note that when treating the fingers for toes, or toes for fingers, you do not need to worry about channel relationships. It is so distal and the image is so powerful that just needling the same spot on the toe to fix the finger will work, regardless of the channel.

The more homologous your images are, the better! Therefore, the radius is the tibia. The ulna is the fibula, etc. The shoulder joint is the hip joint. The edge of the scapula represents the edge of the sacrum. Same for same. You can needle the lower arm for the upper leg. It works. But what is better? The upper arm is *more* like the upper leg. It works much better.

For a better treatment outcome, *expand your images.* Once you are great, you can treat with one needle. So yes, LI 4 will get the face, but do LI 2-3 and Ling gu (you are spreading the image out). Yes, LI 11 will get knee pain, but spread it out, LI 12, LI 11, LI 10, and LI 9. That will make a huge difference in clinical outcomes.

For a better treatment outcome, use *multiple images.*

For headaches, use the toe area as one image, head to feet. Another image is the knee. The knee is the eyes. The shoulder is the head. Three different level images, for the same issue.

Tissue correspondence

For joint pain, needle a joint. For muscle pain, needle a muscle. For tendon pain, needle a tendon. For a vascular issue, needle around a vessel. Why do we like 66.03-4 so much for vascular issues? The dorsalis pedis artery is right there.

Use the "guiding principal," same side channel for pain. Treatment points for back pain on bladder channel? Ling gu, Da bai 22.4-5 with 22.08-09 opposite side. Then same side is BL (BL 65-62-60 awesome "Dao Ma"). Or you could "guide it" with 77.01-2-3-4 (again on the bladder channel same side).

In my experience, I would say that the *homologous structure* is more important than image and channel relationships. Since all channels balance the others to one degree or another, you can be close on your channel relationship and still "get it." However, your image/structure needs to be spot-on for pain.

The tissue correspondence is vastly important as well. You will find that needling the correct tissue type helps you get that last 10–20 percent of pain that your distal needle did not get.

Remember to guide the channel as well. Needle the same side as the pain. Your distal opposite side points will get 90–95 percent of the pain. To get that last 5–10 percent, use the same side channel, with the correct image and correct tissue.

I use these theories every day, on every patient. They will almost always relieve their pain. If I have missed it or it did not work, that would be an exception, and I need to go back and rethink, recheck, re-ask, reanalyze, and use all the other theories (about twenty others) out there. I encourage you to learn all of them.

Internal Disorders

For reaction area and nerve reaction (there is no shortcut—you need a cheat sheet), buy a Dr. Maher book, and make a cheat sheet until you memorize them.

> "**Reaction area**" neurophysical acupuncture. This reflects the knowledge of the delicate energy of the body and the neuroanatomical and neurophysiologic aspects of the body. This acupuncture style also corrects and heals the body through the manipulation of the peripheral and central nervous system by affecting the neuraxis, the actual anatomy, physiology and pathophysiology of the body. (Advanced Tung Style Acupuncture)

Why is the Tung point 44.06 so great for heart issues? It is the cardiac branch nerve. Why are points 77.22-23 so great for the teeth? It is the branch nerve of the teeth. Why is 77.28 great for eyes? It is the optic nerve. Why are points 77.24-25 so great for voice issues? It is the pharynx and larynx nerve, etc.

How about points 11.01-2? LI/SI/6 Fu. Why is the point 44.10 so helpful for leg pain? It is the nerve branch of the legs. Why are points 44.02-3 or 77.01-2-3 effective for spine issues and Du channel issues? It is the reaction area or nerve area of the spine. Point 66.05 is effective for female issues due to the nerve branch of the uterus.

Wu Hu points, 11.27 (1-5), which are the reaction area of the spleen, treat systemic issues such as bony swellings, rheumatoid arthritis, osteoarthritis, traumatic injuries, and damp bi. Points 1010.01+08 help the brain and shaking because of the cerebral nerve branch.

Dao Ma Theory

> "One of most popular Dao Mas and/or Tung points are Ling Gu, Da Bai and Hegu (LI 4). Most, if not all authorities on Tung acupuncture agree that Ling

Gu is located at the junction of the first and second metacarpal bone. Most if not all authorities on Tung agree that Hegu (LI 4) is located in the same area. There is disagreement as to where Da bai is located. Most people suggest that Da bai is located at TCM LI-3, albeit closer to the bone. This Dao Ma is arguably one of the most powerful and significant Dao Mas in the Master Tung system." (Dr. Maher Advanced Tung acupuncture)

What is interesting is that with modern research, we know that the halluces pollicis muscle (the thumb muscle) is one of the densest muscles with one of the highest levels of innervations in the body. This is exactly where this Dao Ma is placed. The quicker we "obtain De Qi," or have an impact on the cerebral cortex, the stronger the healing response will be.

We begin to see the connection of ancient theories and the metaphorical reasons for the power of these points when they match up to modern research. These "Dao Ma" effects are not only witnessed by anecdotal evidence in the clinic every day, but also now via MRIs and neuro-acupuncture research studies.

The significance and power of the Dao Ma is much more than just a simple, "I think it's working." The Dao Ma's have profound healing properties and significant therapeutic results.

"The Dao Ma is holistic in nature in that it frees 'unblocked qi,' treats all organs, frees the San Jiao, harmonizes and regulates all bowels and viscera. It treats the upper, middle, and lower Jiao of the human body with the upper needle, middle needle and lower needle. It affects the "Shen Jing" translated as the nerve. The Dao Ma group will not only treat the TCM perspective, but also the bio medical western perspective of disease. These "nerves" that are part of the Dao Ma treat the actual afferent and efferent nerves of the peripheral and central nervous systems. This ACTUALLY treats the anatomy, physiology, and pathology of the diseased organ or chronic illness." (Dr. Maher Advanced Tung acupuncture)

This is related to Zang fu bei tong relationships with channels. LU/BL TW/KD HT/GB LI/LV, SI/SP, PC/ST. Heart 3 Spirit needles (Dao Ma by Dr. Maher, PC 7-5-4) and 77.08-09 effectively treat stomach, heart, and lung diseases, and digestive, circulation, and respiratory system disorders. Why is this? The PC and ST talk to each other via the

Zang fu bei tong relationships. Remember how you learned in school that PC 6 "empirically" great for digestion?

The five-element concept is a key concept to Master Tung applications. Why is the SPL great for KD reproductive issues/or KD essence issues? Earth controls water. Why is ST so great for asthma? Earth generates metal.

If your problem is internal, do not do the same Dao Ma bilaterally. To treat asthma, assuming it is a lung issue (via the 5 zang line), do not do the 3 scholars, 33.1314-15 bilaterally. Do one arm 33.13-14-15; do the other arm Ling gu, Hegu, Da bai; do one leg 77.08-09-10; do the other leg 88.17-81-19. By doing this, you treat multiple images and multiple channels. You are redundant and overlap your images. In addition, *that makes a huge clinical difference.*

Tung focused a lot on "Western anatomy," such as LU/HT relationships for asthma. Antigen, antibody, and allergies are liver issues. Fatigue is also a liver issue. For headaches not caused by trauma, that is usually hormones. It is often said that "Western medicine was more accepted during Tung's lifetime."

Additional theories to use

Channel relationships: LU/BL, LU/SP, LU/LI, LU/BL, LU/LU LU/LV. I use them all, but as I said, 95 percent of the time I use the three channel relationships for pain: LU/SP for limb pain, LU/BL for torso pain, and LU/LU for guiding the pain and getting that last 5–10 percent of pain.

Twelve segments
Any bone can be broken down into twelve segments. Why is LI 11 so great for dizziness? LI 11 is the "head." The radius is broken down into twelve equal segments: head, neck, upper limbs, lungs, liver, stomach, duodenum, kidney, low back, lower limbs, thigh, foot.

Three Jiaos
Any bone can be broken down into three segments. Why is LI 3/Da bai so great for headaches, and Ling gu so good for back pain? Because LI 3 is the upper jiao, LI 4 the middle jiao, Ling gu the lower jiao.

Time, clock acupuncture

Why bleed from 3–5:00 p.m.? That is Tai yang time. The Tai yang channel has the most blood of any channel. The Tai yang is the best channel to bleed.

Why is Ren 24 so great for neck pain? The Ren, in the front, gets the Du, in the back. It is the same with Ren 24 being on the same line of the C4-5 area.

What we have discovered via modern research is that LI 11 is good for blood pressure. GB 34 is great for systemic pain, depression, and brain problems, such as Parkinson's.

Use the "start of the channel" to fix the "end of the channel" and vice versa. Ren 24 is effective for fertility because it balances Ren 1. The point ST 44 is effective for TMJ and teeth pain because it balances ST 1.

Conclusion on Theories

We can spend the rest of our lives just studying theory. It is great fun. However, in the end, in your clinic, day in and day out, the "rubber needs to meet the road." What good is theory if your patients are not *consistently* getting better? Theory is a guide; it does not always work.

Another acupuncturist said to me, "Brad, all those theories are based from Chinese astrology, the seven heavenly branches and stems, moons and stars and that stuff. You need to study Chinese astrology—that's the truth!" I told him, "That is great. If that is what lights you up, then explain it that way. This is what lights me up. That is how I rationalize my theory. Nobody is right or wrong. That is why it is called theory. The theory I am referring to is what Master Tung taught."

You could forget all of this theory stuff and just memorize everything, but that is boring. Theory is good because it will "direct" you on how to treat. You do not need points; there really are no points, such as doing "reverse" hand/Su Jok/Koryo hand acupuncture. The theory will guide you to your choice and help you when you are confused or lost. However, clinical experience will show us if it works or not. That is the power of Master Tung acupuncture—backed by amazing, rich theory, and proven by Master Tung and his teachers/students.

How do I communicate to my patients?

We are setting the stage on the neuro-endocrine stage tissue repair and endorphin release, which in itself lowers inflammation and causes tissues to repair. This puts us in a parasympathetic mode, where tissue replacement increases. There is also an increase in secretion of endorphins, which lowers cortisol. The needles will release local and global anti-inflammatories in your body, such as "Beta Endorphin" which is about 200 times stronger than morphine.

Blood Tests Prove It

The four things that we can prove via blood tests that acupuncture does are:

- Repair damaged tissue and create new healthy tissue
- Modulate your neuro endocrine system
- Vasodilate your injured body part
- Reduce swelling in the nerve endings that keep sending pain signals to the brain

That is what I tell my patients. But you should do whatever lights you up. Figure out how you want to say it. What motivates you? Communicate that.

Clinic Notes

- I use 34-36 gauge needles, MAC single needles.
- I have patients sit for thirty minutes with the needles. I tell them they should feel better *today*, right now, if I did my job right. However, please give me two to four treatments so that we can see how you are doing. We determine what percentage of the pain we relieved.
- Are you responding and healing?
- After a few treatments, I can give you a straight-up answer if I can help, how much I can help, and what it will take (i.e., acupuncture, herbs, diet, lifestyle).

In my experience, the most consistent and reliable results you will attain with patients will be as follows.

1. Find the most homologous structure; this is your image/mirror.

2. If you are treating limb pain, use *system one* (LU/SP, etc.). On the torso use *system four* (clock opposite Dr. Tan) or Tung Zang fu bei tong.
3. If you are treating internal disorders, use your reaction area, 5 Element concept, or Zang fu paired organ systems.
4. To improve your results, use the correct tissue, bone for bone, etc.
5. To improve your clinical outcomes, use multiple images, multiple theories, and spread your images.
6. In the beginning you will need more than five to six needles; as you get better, you can use fewer and fewer needles.

Finally, we all need to walk our own path. You will need to practice, in real life on real patients and make real mistakes. You will learn, you will fail, you will relearn and rethink and retry. *We are all students forever.* Chinese medicine has been "dynamic" not "static" for 3,000 years. We need to practice, critically think, and practice some more.

The glory is in the attempt. If you have questions, please e-mail me. I hope this helps shed light on the difficulty of "Master Tung" acupuncture. As Einstein said, "If you can't explain it in a simple way, you don't understand it well enough."

CHAPTER 4

WHERE DOES DISTAL TUNG ACUPUNCTURE FALL SHORT?

There is an old saying, "You can't be all things to all people all the time." Master Tung acupuncture, though famous and impressive, is therapeutically no different. There are certain types of patients and conditions that are challenging to treat.

Tinnitus

In my experience, although many books say certain points are effective for tinnitus, I honestly think body points are too "hit and miss" for me to say I can effectively and consistently treat tinnitus in my clinic. I have seen better results with ear acupuncture. I have successfully treated tinnitus with Tung points, but to me it seemed anecdotal in the sense that I cannot predict how it will work. I prefer to use herbs as the main modality for tinnitus.

Shoulder Pain

I see many practitioners struggle with shoulder pain using a distal method. In my opinion, the reason for that is that the best homologous relationship is the hip. But in America, typically we do not needle the hip because it is around the groin and buttock area. This being said, we need to pick another "image." Most people pick the wrist or the ankle. Yes, we can pick the mid lower leg, the hand, and also treat the healthy shoulder. There are many other ideas.

Still, the *best* relationship to treat the shoulder is the hip. If we are not able to use the best relationship, in my opinion the best points for shoulder pain are Fan hou jue (on the thumb) and 77.09, which is basically ST 38. These points never cease to amaze me.

I think the reason they are not used as much is that these two images—the knuckle of the thumb is the shoulder, and the mid lower leg is the shoulder—are not so easy to see. I do frequently use the wrist and ankle for the shoulder, but I can always rely on Fan hou jue and 77.09 as my reliable pain points for the shoulder. These points are also so wonderful because they treat any type and any channel for shoulder pain, which most points do not.

The other issue with hips and shoulders is that they are both limbs, and they are part of your torso. There are so many different attachments and muscles going on it can be hard to distinguish exactly where or why they hurt, thus making your treatment ineffective.

Upper Neck

Upper neck and shoulder are probably the biggest hurdles or stumbling blocks for acupuncturists. Most, if not all, Americans have neck and shoulder pain. It is chronic in nature and complex in the fact that it involves a lot of different muscles, bones, tendons. It is typically repeatedly aggravated by life and/or work.

Patients also usually come to see us as a last resort. I think only 3 percent or less of my patients use me as a "first responder." I am always this provider: "Well, I tried everything else, and nothing else has worked. Why not try acupuncture?"

The only people I treat as a "first responder" are my patients who originally came in and said, "I'll only see you as the last resort," they got better, and now they use me as a primary care provider.

Chronic neck and shoulders can be difficult to treat due to all the channels that cross in the upper neck. The biggest challenge is to determine which muscles are involved. To compare, the bladder channel is used for more acute issues. The kidney controls the deeper muscles for more chronic issues.

The triple warmer controls the posterior scalene, a very common muscle involved in upper neck pain, but many people do not think to treat the posterior scalene. The small intestine controls the levator scapula, which is almost always indicated in stress-induced neck and shoulder pain.

The thing that confuses most people is that the rhomboids are superficially controlled by the small intestine channel, but really the large intestine is what we need to balance, according to the muscle tendino channels.

The large intestine channel is often overlooked in the treatment of the back. The large intestine channel is also responsible for the subscapularis, which most people do not think of.

Another tricky one is the supraspinatus, which is controlled by the triple warmer. The triple warmer also runs to the posterior shoulder, though one would think that this area is posterior to the location of SI 9 and SI 10. *TW*

Back and neck pain can be a challenge with the Du, kidney, bladder, triple warmer, small intestine, and large intestine all possibly needing treatment, and yes, to some extent, the gall bladder. I know most people are saying, "Wait a minute ... the gall bladder is all over the upper neck. What about the gall bladder?"

TREAT BL for GB

In my experience, yes, the gall bladder affects the upper neck. The best way to treat that is usually the bladder. The bladder controls the whole trap and SCM. The gall bladder is also there, but in my experience, a greater portion of pain and irritation will be resolved by treating the bladder instead of the gall bladder. You can see this if you look at the muscle tendino channels. I do treat both to cover my bases, but usually treating the GB and focusing on the GB and where it goes will not give the relief that is needed.

I have noticed with back pain that narrowing of the foramen is extremely difficult—if not impossible—to treat. This is always seen in the elderly who do not hurt until they walk about twenty feet and then feel better only if they sit down. That is how I usually see narrowing of the foramen in my patients. I find that yes, we can give relief, but to actually heal the patient is very difficult.

Response in Three to Four Visits is the Norm, with an 80 percent Improvement Immediately

I have also noticed that patients who do not respond to distal treatment in three to four visits will rarely respond if you continue to treat them. I have had a few patients who did not respond after three to four visits but did respond around the tenth. That is the exception, however, and not the rule. *Typically, I look for a patient to have 80 percent or better pain relief on the table when I treat them.* That is what I call a successful result.

Obviously, we try for 100 percent, and that does happen more often than not, but as long as I achieve an 80 percent reduction in pain, my patients and I are very happy.

With distal (Tung) acupuncture, your patient should feel better about two to five seconds after the needles are inserted. Even with internal issues, if they have obvious symptoms, such as breathing problems, or gastric issues, we will see an immediate improvement. If I am not able to discern if they are better or not, I suggest two treatments for two weeks. We can assess over the ten to fourteen days how they are doing. It is at this point that I discuss with the patient what our next steps are.

Heat and Cold

When patients tell you that heat or cold affects them, that is one of the best signs for a good treatment outcome. When they say, "No matter what, hot or cold, nothing ever changes my pain or condition," those patients are very hard to treat. You can do local on them and not worry about inflammation or irritation, but the clinical outcomes are hard to predict for these people.

Of the patients who say, "Cold makes it worse, and heat makes it better," 100 percent of those people will respond extremely well to any treatment, distal or local. The patients who say, "Heat makes it worse, or I feel worse at the end of the day," will not do well with local because of the swelling; they will do better with distal needles.

Use Enough Needles

In my experience, the biggest challenge acupuncturists face when doing imaging and mirroring in the beginning is they do not use enough needles to cover the whole image/mirror and/or to cover all the channels.

For instance, when you treat the upper back, you can cover all the back channels with Ren 24, HT 7-6-5-4 inserted from the SI channel to the HT channel. Three weights, 77.05-6-7, Seven tigers 77.26, and SP 5.5-6, LV 5-6. If that does not clear it, you can add LI or ST. So you can see how you can use just a few channels to treat all the channels

double saint on lung channel
double child

You can fix the upper back with 22.01-2 and Ren 24. That is for a specific pain condition; it will not result in a great treatment outcome if a patient has pain all over their upper neck and upper back. I agree that it is best to use a few needles, but in my experience, it is more important to heal the patient.

If these patients with neck and upper back pain actually came to us when they first experienced the pain, then I agree that a few simple needles here or there would fix them. When your patient has long-term chronic pain in the neck and shoulder, you can be sure multiple channels, multiple muscles, multiple discs, and multiple bones will be involved.

You could do just two or three needles per treatment and expect your patients to come back three times a week for two months. When I am overseas, I can cure type 2 diabetes with acupuncture alone. But you must treat three times a week for two months. This is usually not possible in America. You need to fix the patient *today*. We are a "fast-food nation," and unfortunately, all our patients are from "Missouri" (the Show-Me State). They need and expect results, right now. That is one of the most rewarding aspects of using the Tung system—you *do* get results immediately.

I know some people say you cannot do two channels with one needle. I find that inaccurate in the clinical setting. I often use one needle to treat two channels. The body does not know if you are needling from the dorsal or the ventral side. It does not know if you are needling from anterior to posterior, or vice versa. What does it know? It knows a small metal filament is stimulating a nerve node. After you stimulate one nerve node, you can insert deeper and stimulate another node. I use this technique all the time in my clinic.

I have also heard that you cannot treat pain bilaterally since that will be too many needles and/or the "wave" of the needles going through the body will cancel each other out. This is not correct in a clinical setting. I regularly treat bilateral pain with the same needles bilaterally, and the needles do not cancel each other out.

Yes, I have heard the expression of "no free lunch." The next time you needle Ling gu, first insert your needle into Ling gu. Then ask your patient if her back pain is gone. She will usually say yes. If this patient also has upper neck pain, you can angle the Ling gu needle into 22.02, one of the points of the double saint and double child. Then ask her if her upper back is better. She will say yes. She will not say yes, that her upper back pain is gone, *until* your needle passes through Ling gu and hits the nerve node at 22.02.

Another example is 66.04, Hou zhu. I use that a lot for stress, somewhat like the four gates in TCM. If you insert the needle and wait five minutes, most likely they will be less stressed. If they had an eye issue, that needle will not treat it. However, you can then extend the needle down into 55.02, flower bone one. It is on the underside of 66.04. You can extend the needle at 66.04 into the nerve node at 55.02, and the patient will report that their eye issues are better. The list is endless.

In my experience, you can needle from one point to another, and as long as you are touching both nerve nodes, the body will respond. The body does not know you are using one needle for two channels.

This whole imaging and mirroring is not even really a Tung thing. We image and mirror every day in TCM; we just do not call it that. The TCM point, GB 41, the Dai mai, helps with mid-section issues. That point is not in the mid-section.

The TCM point SP 6 is used for gynecological issues; it is not in the groin. TCM point ST 36 is used for fatigue, but it is not in the spleen. SP 4 is used for digestive problems, but it is not in the stomach. LI 4 is the master point of the face, yet it is in the hand. TCM point GB 39 treats neck pain, but it is in the leg.

TCM uses BL 40 for low back pain, but it is in the leg. So, mirroring and imaging are *a part of all acupuncture*, not just Tung! It is not a new or exclusive idea. The idea was used and made famous in Tung acupuncture. You could say that Tung acupuncture developed the theory that *explains* mirror and image. Tung acupuncture developed theories, but it is not a new idea to all of acupuncture.

I always suggest to students when learning Tung points or TCM points to get away from the words "distal" or "local." I do not really care. The only thing I am concerned with is that the points are reliable. Are the points reliable? Are they effective, consistent, and miraculous? Yes? Then, let us use them. I say to use what works and get rid of the rest. A system of not having a system, a "way" that has "no way," this is my way.

The two things that always amazed me in Tung acupuncture is the lack of points for stress and insomnia. There are only about seven points and six points respectively that have indications of "stress and/or insomnia." Master Tung's system has over 740 points. That is less than 1 percent of his fabulous system that is dedicated to stress or sleep. Does this mean Master Tung acupuncture does not treat stress or sleep? Of course not. We just have to do a bit of deductive reasoning.

He has many points for conditions we do not even see any more. How many times have you seen cholera in your clinic? This is a disease that comes from bacteria from bad water or uncooked food. Diseases, and thus the points used to treat them, are conditions and reflections of the time in society.

In Master Tung acupuncture, there are many points for scarlet fever, tuberculosis, and polio. Why is this? Is it that Master Tung cared more about these conditions than stress or sleep? No, it is not. It is the same reason our classical texts do not have a lot on cancer (though it was around back then and there is a bit of writings on it), and there is no information on type 2 diabetes. It did not exist back then. Type 1, wasting and thirsting syndrome in our classics, did exist, but not type 2.

It was not until people ate large amounts of junk food and other unhealthy foods that people in large parts of the world became so overweight. Even in America, there was no childhood type 2 diabetes before 1980. This is the same reason why Master Tung had such a low number of points for sleep and stress. I really do not think he saw much of it.

From 1900 to the 1970s, China and Taiwan were not first-world countries. They were mostly rural. I have treated tens of thousands of rural people. These people work hard! They work in fields; they work in manual labor. At the end of the day, they are tired! I always say, I never met a farmer who could not sleep. They are up early, they work hard all day, and at the end of the day, they sleep well.

I would think most of the 400,000 patients Master Tung saw fell into the same category. This is why we see such a small number of points indicated for sleep problems. Stress is much the same. Stress is a "rich country" problem. This means that food, shelter, and safety are taken care of (see Maslow's pyramid), and now you and I have so much time on our hands to ponder life. We get depressed because our Facebook pictures are not as cool as our friends' Facebook pictures.

We get stressed because our friend's car is nicer than ours. None of this matters when we are trying to find food, shelter, or safety. When I was in India, I treated only a few cases of depression out of 8,000. A few! In America, if I treat 8,000 people, I would bet at least 6,000 would have depression as a secondary concern. At least 2,000–3,000, would have depression as the major complaint. We are a nation of worried, stressed, and sad individuals where about one in ten takes an antidepressant. But more alarmingly, there has been a 400 percent increase in people reporting depression.

If Master Tung were alive today, I can almost guarantee he would have more points for treating depression since it is such a common disease in society today. This is why you see many "older" diseases in his textbooks, such as polio (almost eradicated now), scarlet fever (I treated that only two times in my whole career), and tuberculosis (I have treated this only overseas).

The question remains, is Master Tung acupuncture good for stress and sleep? Yes, of course it is. We just do not have any empirical points such as an An Mian (TCM point). We know with An Mian (peaceful sleep) that this point lights up the sleep center of the brain, and via MRI scans the sleep center is balanced.

In Master Tung acupuncture, we need to treat the root. A few insomnia causes can be a weak liver, heat in the heart, blood stagnation, anemia, pain, or hormone imbalances. We can treat those causes and thus cure the sleeping problem. Patient problems could be rooted in hormone issues, pain, dampness, and/or spleen and stomach issues (where 90 percent of serotonin is made).

When it comes to sleep and stress, remember it is not that Tung does not have those points; it is that I suspect he rarely saw those problems. I certainly never do, unless I am treating in Western cultures.

CHAPTER 4

LETTERS TO BRAD – YOUR QUESTIONS ANSWERED

Brad has been answering questions about Tung acupuncture for several years. He invites everyone to send him questions. These answers are very brief. He answers these questions between patients, so he wants to be clear that he has not elaborated to the extent he would for a case study. However, the letters give him the chance to address a wide variety of problems. The names and other identifying facts have been removed.

List of cases

Achilles tendon pain
Bulging disc, back pain, and pinched nerve
Can you combine Tung with TCM?
Dizziness in older people is damp and phlegm
Dysmenorrhea-Tung style
How to treat your own hip pain
Inguinal hernia
Low back pain treated using homologous scapula
Man fell on carpet, now has neck pain
Meniere's, tinnitus, and dizziness
Menstrual cycles and fertility timing
Mixing Chinese and Japanese, setting up for failure?
Nocturnal enuresis in a ten-year-old boy
Parkinson's
Post herpetic neuralgia
Quick fix for calming people
Restless leg syndrome
Severe sciatica in Australia
Varicose veins

Achilles Tendon Pain

Good morning Brad,

Thank you so much for all the wonderful information you shared with us all this past weekend. This was the first course I took with both eLotus and with you, and I thoroughly enjoyed the class. I have already been using many of the techniques you taught, in my clinic with great success.

I have a question regarding sharp pain along the Achilles. If the pain is on the actual Achilles tendon, starting at the base of the heel, to about two inches above the malleolus, which channel do you use to base the treatment (UB/KD)? As this is on the limbs, I would think to use either SI or HT. I used several points near the wrist around the ulnar tendon, combined with the Shu stream points on the KD and UB with minimal success.

Do you have any other possible suggestions? Also, is heel pain considered a kidney channel issue?

Brad:

Yes, I would say the heel is the kidney. If it is between the channels, then needle between the channels. It sounds like you are doing it right.
If it is right on the Achilles tendon, needle right into the ulnar tendon, all the way down to the pisiform. That is how I usually treat it.

Bulging Disc, Back Pain, and Pinched Nerve

Hi Brad,

Have you ever treated a bulging disc/pinched nerve successfully, or do you often find that you'll need to refer out?

Brad: Yes, although it can be difficult, I have success with disc problems. Sometimes you cannot help, but that is rare.

Question: My dad has been experiencing intense lumbago upon extension, so I'd say bulging disc is my working diagnosis. I tried all my lumbago points (Ling gu, Da bai, SI 3, Shen guan, mirrored points via Tan's method), but nothing is touching it.

Brad: I would agree with you; those points do not work for me very often. What I like to do for this problem is to do a superficial needle and slide it down the external occipital protuberance (EOP) on the back of the head; this is the Tung point 1010.25. It is located in the area of DU 18. Start in that area with a 1.5-inch needle and slide it down so it hits the EOP. That will get the Du portion of the pain. That is very important if it is disc pain because the root of it is on the Du channel.

Then do the three upright tendons. On the LI channel, go to LI 11, then go two cun up the LI channel; that is your first point. Then two more cun up the arm is the second point. Then go two more cun up; that is your third point. Make sure it is on the LI channel and make sure your needle "taps" the bone, the humerus, with a perpendicular insertion. They are called Gu ci yi, Gu ci er, and Gu ci san. These points are used for bone for bone treatments. LI balances KD and it is also the reaction of the Du meridian.

On the other arm, treat the shoulder. Do the points TW 14, SI 14, and LI 15, and Pian Jian (Tung point). Just find deep points in the shoulder area and insert the needle deep into the joint. I prefer points toward the SI and TW areas. I will even needle into the lateral edge of the scapula; again, you need to make sure you tap the lateral edge of the scapula and/or get the needle deep into the shoulder joint. The shoulder joint is SI/L5 joint. The scapula is the sacrum.

On the legs, do GB 31, Tung 88.25, and tap the bone. Use a two-inch needle if necessary. Treating just one leg is fine. Tung point 88.25 is the number one point for pain, and in the Ling shu the GB controls bone as well. So TCM says kidney is bone, and Ling Shu says GB gets bone. I treat both to cover my bases.

On the feet, treat KI 2, 3, 7, and on the other foot, BL 60, 62, 65. And again, insert one or two needles into the deep joint space of the lateral malleolus.

I agree that Ling gu, Da bai, and SI 3 will not usually get this type of problem. I just had a patient who had six surgeries on her back in the L5/S1 area. She had disc problems, laminectomies, and all types of other issues. She was in excruciating pain. After two weeks, with treatment three times a week, then two more weeks with treatment twice a week, she is pain free and is no longer taking any medication. We focused on the shoulder to treat the hip, the upper arm to treat the back. I did use all the San chas, Yi er San, which are basically the TCM Yao tongs, a few times. I also used a lot of KD and BL points at the knee and feet. Points: KD 10, 3, BL 40, 65-62-60.

Just do not forget the Du; that is the one channel most people forget. They always focus on the GB, KD, and BL. The Du is super important. If you need to, you can treat the belly points (the front will treat the back). That works great if nothing else is working.

Can you Combine Tung with TCM?

Hi Brad,

I'm currently starting to watch your courses on Dr. Tung on elotus.org and I had one quick question as I'm still confused. Can you combine TCM points with Dr. Tung points? For example, if I'm treating shoulder pain and want to use Dr. Tung's points (which I believe one combination is Sanzhong?), can I use traditional points like four gates to move blood, etc. and throw in Sanzhong?

It looks like lots of Master Tung teachers mention that it is considered poor acupuncture in their lectures that I skimmed through, but I can't reason why. Since I'm proficient in TCM, but it doesn't always work for certain conditions, I want to be able to combine, but have no idea if that lessens the treatment results. Would you have some time to provide insight? Thank you in advance for your time and consideration.

Brad: Yes, everyone has his own opinion.

I do NOT usually do TCM with Tung needles. I do about, 98 percent Tung needles. If a patient requests TCM points or something they have had before, I give them what they ask for, as long as they get better.

I have treated over 50,000 people. The reason I say you can combine Tung and TCM is that 99 percent of the people who want to learn Tung needles already do TCM. And they do TCM in their practice to make money and earn a living. What would happen if they did only Tung needles and got no results? They would go out of business. So I always say, start distal, do Tung needles, ask the patient how he/she feels. If the patient feels better, then stop. If you missed it or feel afraid that you did not get results, then go ahead and add in your TCM needles.

Really, does the "body" know what you are doing? Does the "body" know if it is a distal, or local, or five-element or Tung points? NO, IT DOES NOT. It knows that you are stimulating something; whether it is local or distal, or Tung or TCM is irrelevant to your body.

I say heal the body with whatever needle works. The reason you DO NOT want to do Tung and TCM (local) is that they both heal by DIFFERENT mechanisms. Sometimes that does not matter (for example, with asthma). You can do Ren 17, LU 1, LU 2 and Tung points, and it works great.

But sometimes, with pain patients, if you do a distal needle that heals a certain way and THEN A LOCAL needle that causes inflammation, that usually will not work. They can cancel each other out. It is not because the body says TCM and Tung do not work together, but because the healing mechanisms differ.

But I always say to use it together so that new people can use Tung and TCM together, continue to learn, help people, and not go out of business. This way you can get good at Tung points, use your TCM when needed, and be happy. A great example is back pain.

TCM people treat the patient lying facedown, with their back exposed. *Before* you treat the sacrum, treat Tung 1010.25 (assuming they have low back pain). The Tung point 1010.25 is on the back of the head, so your patient is in a *perfect* position. Let your patient breathe for five seconds and ask him/her, "Is your back better?" It should be. If it is, then stop; do some massage or something, no local needles. You fixed it.

But if you ask them and they say, "Yeah, my back still hurts," well, you learned something. Now that 1010.25 did not give you the results you wanted, you can learn, research, and study why you missed it. Then go ahead and do your local TCM needles. Everybody wins. You have learned something, and your patient still heals. How can that be poor acupuncture? Good luck!

Dysmenorrhea treatment – Tung Style

Hi Brad,

Question: I have a question for you about Tung style for dysmenorrhea. I think I found the protocol below in the Evergreen clinical manual under Mense-Ease, but I can't remember. Anyway, I have used it with very good success with lots of women. The thing is, I have no idea why it works. Would you mind explaining to me why these points work for dysmenorrhea? I'm so curious!

Right: LU 5, 6, 7, ST 36, GB 41, 42
Left: LI 4, Ling gu, SP 9, 8, 6,

Brad: There are many reasons as to why and how, but I will do my best to explain the reason why this works.

What channels run through the menstrual area? The liver, stomach, gall bladder, spleen, kidney, and Ren. But one thing that was not addressed here is the Ren channel. I would add in yin tang, Du 26, Du 20. The Du treats the Ren, the Du treats Du, and the images of the other points are the menstrual area.

In addition, the LU will balance the KD and SP. For the image, LU 5, 6, 7, images the lower abdomen. The wrist is the pelvis. LU 7 is also the Master/Key/Confluent Point of Ren mai.

For ST 36, the stomach treats the stomach, and the stomach also treats the spleen. I would argue that the "yang ming," regardless of the channel, will treat jue yin. Liver is jue yin. ST 36 is the earth point on earth channel, so it builds blood. Also, ST 36 is the belly-button area on stomach.

GB 41-42 is the lower pelvis area like Ren 2-3-4 area. GB gets GB, GB treats LV, GB is bone as per Ling shu, master point of Dai mai, shu stream point, moves the liver qi, GB 41 and 42 are coupled points to make a stronger effect, like a "Dao Ma" Tung idea. Two points are as strong as three points; you get a synergistic effect.

For LI 4, the LI gets ST, LI gets LV, and LI gets KD. Point LI 4 is in the middle of bone, so it is the middle of the body. LI is probably the best for gynecological issues because of those relationships, LV, KD, ST, it clears it all.

Ling gu is at the metatarsal, so it is the lower Jiao. LI 4 is middle Jiao, and Ling gu is lower Jiao. And again, LI gets KD, LV, ST.

For SP 9-8-6, SP gets SP, SP gets ST. The image of the lower leg, just like Lung, the lower arm is the lower abdomen. So SP is the belly-button area, SP 8 is like the Ren 6 area, and SP 6 is like Ren 3-4 area. SP 6 is the three leg yin point. In Five Elements, the earth, the spleen, balances the water, the kidney. Reproductive issues are the kidney.

There is more to it, but from a Tung perspective, that should help. I like to focus on LI, ST, SP, LV and LU as well when I treat. It balances all the channels that run through the abdomen.

How to Treat Your Own Hip Pain

Hi Brad,

I hope this message finds you well. I just finished watching your webinar from Elotus: Essential Tung's Acupuncture: Clinical Strategies for Treating Pain. I currently practice some basic Tung points and they work well for me. I am new to Tung's method and I love it.

However, my question to you is I need to learn how to treat myself. Here is my problem: I started getting hip pain in December and by January, I have radiculopathy down my left leg to my foot. I got an X-ray that revealed degeneration at L5-S1 and possible bulges and herniations at L3-L4.

Some arthritis was noticed and some narrowing at the facet joints too. I understand an MRI will only reveal the nature of the discs, but due to the radiculopathy, it's what I am thinking.

The pain goes down to my foot and it moves a lot, changing from GB/ST/UB, but the main problem is I feel like I have a knife in my left hip joint. The X-ray also revealed my right pelvis is rotated forward, so my SI joint is out and I can't get it back in.

I've tried chiropractic, which makes it worse, and massage, and I've been to four different acupuncturists with no success. No disrespect to them, but I feel the acupuncturists were missing something. I'm using an inversion table now and it seems to be helping a little bit.

I am stretching, meditating, you name it. I think the trigger started when I was taking 16 credits online last semester because I was sitting way too much.

I am having a hard time finding a good acupuncturist to treat back pain/radiculopathy, as I just moved to Florida a couple of years ago. Do you have any suggestions for me as far as treatments I can do on myself? I really think treating around the scapula would be beneficial for me, but I can't get to some of those points.

I was just wondering if you have any tricks up your sleeve on how to treat yourself! This is slowing me down, and I need to get back on track. Any info you can give me would be greatly appreciated. Thanks for sharing your knowledge on Master Tung acupuncture!

Also, what herbs from Evergreen would you recommend? Thanks again for your help! I feel like the shoe-shine girl with the dirty shoes—helping everyone else but can't help myself!

Brad: I love what you said, a shoe-shine girl with ugly shoes ... LOVE IT. :-)

Regarding treating yourself, this is why I got into acupuncture. This is what I used on myself EVERY DAY until I got better. I was supposed to get surgery for a blown-out disc on L5/S1, and I had radiating pain into my toes! I could not sneeze, poop, pee, walk, have sex ... NOTHING! It was horrible!

So, first off, bleed yourself every three weeks. Find BL 40 and bleed any distended vein about two inches above, below, and to the right or the left.

Get in the shower, get an 18-gauge needle, a razor or lancet, and bleed those veins. I would do that every three to four weeks. If you do not like bleeding, that's cool. Do not do it.

Acupuncture points:

Yao tong points. These points are at the base of five fingers.
Basically, Ling gu, SI 4, in that zone
All five finger joints, opposite side
33.12, 1.5 cun distal to SI8, opposite side
LI 12 opposite side
44.02-3-4 opposite side (look those points up)

Same side:

BL 40-65
GB 34, 41
GB 31

Distal Imaging

Ear points, at the sacrum area

1010.19-20 on your face, bilateral
1010.22, Bi yi on your nose opposite side

Opposite side, KD 2-3-4--7, 10

Those should all work.

Lct me know if you are not getting better. I hope that helps.

Hi Brad: You're the man! Thanks so much for your quick response. I too got into acupuncture for similar reasons. I will give those points a shot and bleed BL 40. I should have done that a while ago. Thanks a million times for your help. I'll keep you posted.

Brad: PLEASE! Yes, if this does not work, let me know. I have more things you can try. Do about ten of those points. You can pick or choose, whatever floats your boat.

I would change up the points to confuse the body, and keep it guessing.

Inguinal Hernia

Dear Brad,

What are your favorite points for inguinal hernia? I have not treated it for a while, so I am a little rusty. I remember LI 16 area in the opposite shoulder joint worked well last time I treated it.

Brad: The best points are on the ulnar side of the first metacarpal. Tung points 11.01-2, 3, 4 are great Tung points for hernias.

Low back pain –treated using homologous scapula

Dear Brad:

I have been watching your most recent webinar on elotus and once again it's great! Fantastic Job!

My question is regarding treating low back pain. I really like the concept of using the scapula as a homologous structure. I've been using Lung 1, 2 area for the past couple of years with good results. My question is how do you get up from the SI joint and higher into the lumbar area with this image? It seemed like you were indicating the rhomboids, but since there's really no "up" from the scapula unless you get into the neck and head, I just couldn't get how to approach the common L2-L5 pain.

Brad: Yes, that is a good question and I agree, I did not really do a great job explaining that. When I got done with the seminar, I realized that I did not really explain that all that well.

To treat L2-5 pain, I really like the Yao tongs, all five of them. I then add in the humerus. I like TW 14 and SI 11 in particular. That is on the shoulder joint, or is it TW 15 and SI 12? I am sorry; I forgot the TCM points. But I like those two points to treat L5 pain. The humerus is the femur, and the posterior aspect where it connects to the scapula is the L5/S1 joint. The lateral edge of the patella is the lateral edge of the sacrum. SI 10 would be very close TCM point for the L5/S1 joint space.

Another favorite of mine is that 44.01 Dao Ma by Maher, basically, LI 12 (tap the bone), then 2 cun proximal, and 2 cun proximal. Or it is called Gu Cu yi er san.

You can also just hang the arms, and where the arms cross the sacrum, needle those points. I then take the mid arm image to the leg. I do about three needles at KI 8-9-

10, and the area of BL 40, 2 cun distal, 2 cun distal. This is not my favorite way to do things, but it does work.

Also, do not forget about 44.02-3-4; they are great Master Tung points. Go 2 cun up from LI 11, 3 cun up from LI 11, and 4 cun up from LI 11, then go between the LI and TW channels. Angle in between the channels and hit the back side of the humerus.

On the head, I love threading one needle, 1.5 cun. It is 1010.25. Start about 1 cun above the EOP, and thread down the EOP. It works like a charm. I love that point. Remember, the EOP is the L5, so go a little above it and there should be L2. But I find L2 just above the EOP. That is theory versus my experience.

For the hand, if you do not do the Yao tongs, do the San cha yi er san. Basically thread the needle from the PIP joint into the base of the metatarsals.

You can always treat L5/S1 on the ear as well. The points are right around the shen men area. The patient will most likely have some mark around the L5/S1 zone on the back.

Do not forget your usual points, the KD 3, BL 40, SI 3, BL 65 and the old and faithful, Ling gu.

But be sure to put five needles up in the SI 10 shoulder area, and you should get it.

One of my no-brainer back treatments is, if the back hurts on the left at the typical low back spot, like L5/S1, I will needle all three San cha, yi er san with Ling gu and SI 4 or a modified SI4 (might switch out SI4 for 22.08-09) and might switch out the san chas for 11.11-12.

Then at the elbow, I use 33.12, heart gate, and usually Gu Cu yi er san. (I like it because it treats LI for KD, the image is good, and it is the reaction area of the Du.) Then I will use SI 10, TW 14 and LI 15 (pian jian).

For the arm, I have three different images going on and all sorts of reaction areas, channel relationships, and expanded images. I want to cover any and everything on the back. On the same side, I use BL 65-40, GB 43-34, or if needed, 88.25. That usually gets it.

Sometimes I will trade out those points and focus more on the same side lateral malleolus, which is great for hip and back pain. The image is amazing, and the channel relationships are perfect. And although most people think of it for neck pain, it is great for low and mid to low back pain, Tung 77.01-2-3. I also really like that 77.03-4 for the L2, L1, T12-10 stuff, so do not forget those.

Question: I would say that helps a whole lot! I'm psyched to work more of these points in. I feel like I was knocking it out of the park on back pain and then lately just got a slew of patients who haven't been getting those amazing results. I'm printing your email out and putting it in my little book of pearls! I appreciate your contribution immensely. I will let you know how it works on my patients.

Brad: That sounds good! Yes, I find that with back patients you have to be flexible. I will get ten patients with the same issue, I use the same points, and I get results. Then, that eleventh patient comes in with the same problem. I use the same points and get no results! Back pain is TRICKY! And medicine is so humbling. That is why I gave so many combinations.

I also like the finger spine points, 11.10-11, down the dorsum side of middle finger, i.e., the middle finger is the spine.

I also like the three-point combo, BL 65-62-60. It is a Dao Ma by Maher, and it is a very good combination.

Do not forget, some very powerful points for the back are needling into the tummy. Just find the exact side on the tummy and needle that. The front gets back. It works well. Sometimes that will be the only thing that gets it. With back pain, you have to be flexible.

Man fell on carpet, and now has neck pain

Dear Brad:

A man in his sixties fell back on carpet and experienced a whiplash-like effect. He had neck stiffness, but now, a few months later, it is a sharp throbbing pain starting at the left side of his neck radiating and up above the skull. The pain also goes down the left side of his face and into his eye. He's gone to see the doctors and did MRIs, CTs, X-rays, and they can't find anything wrong with him.

I've never been really good at head pain. I haven't mastered it yet since I don't see a lot of people with headaches and migraines.

I am thinking that Circulation SJ might do him some good. But he might not be ready for herbs right now.

The points I am considering are Shen guan, LV 2, upright tendons on the right side, and some Ashi points. But how do you image the face on the hands? Where are the eyes? Do you have any treatment ideas for me?

Brad: That type of pain is very common. It is typically the GB 20 area that is radiating up over the head into the eyes.

For that neck pain, I like Flex Spur at 40% + Ge gen tang 40% + Flex SC at 20%. That is great. That is an almost 100 percent guarantee. If it does not work, add in Back HD because there is swelling, disc issues. You can take out the Flex SC and do the Back HD formula.

For points, I would do:

Same side GB 43-42-41 and deep in the joint space of GB 40, GB 34

Same side, BL 65-64-63-62-60

Opposite side, LV 2-3, 8

Same side, SP 3-4-9

On the hand, all opposite side:
A 5 so jing dians, so basically LI 3, Lou zhen, so jing dian, TW 3, SI 3 and same side San cha san.

I can give you Tung points, but it is easier and quicker if I just say the TCM points. Does that help? That will totally nail it—trust me. Oh, and add in Ren 24. The front, Ren, will get the back, Du.

Meniere's, Tinnitus, and Dizziness

Hi Brad,

I watched the webinar this morning. Thank you. I am a newbie. I just got my license in February of this year.

I have a patient and would appreciate your opinion regarding his treatment. He is a 66-year-old man with Meniere's disease and tinnitus. It is a chronic condition. It started five years ago following a cardiac incident after which he needed a pacemaker inserted. He has a constant buzzing in his left ear. Tongue: body looks pale and is swollen with thick white coat. From TCM point of view, I think there is a pattern of internal wind with phlegm damp. He is not really having any kidney symptoms (low back pain or urinary problems).

For the first and second treatment, I used KI 3, ST 40, SP 9, bilateral SI 3, SJ 17, SI 19, SI 17 on the affected side, SJ 5 and GB 43 on unaffected side.

After another Tung seminar, I changed track and used Master Tung points Three yellow bilateral, Ling gu and PC 6 on the left and LI 11 and GB 43 on right.

I saw him today, did the same points as above, but added SJ 17 and SI 19 on the left, and bled his ear apex at end of the treatment. The problem is he is not getting any better. His tongue looks better, but he is still getting attacks of vertigo, and yesterday he had one that took two hours to settle.

What do you think? Of course there are lots of points I can use, but how many is too many and at what point should I stop treating if we are not seeing an improvement?

Brad: Thanks for watching, and those are great questions.
First off, is your patient improving? I usually treat patients four to six times. If they do not improve, I tell them, "You might get better. If you want to continue, we can. We might get lucky, but I usually see some improvement by now, and it worries me that we are not seeing any yet."

Yes, ear problems in older people can be difficult to treat. Any ear issue is difficult to treat with acupuncture alone. Most acupuncturists will have a 50 percent success rate with this problem. Since it is damp and phlegm, it is much easier to treat. I think local acupuncture is great, with Ling gu, San cha san, Three emperors, the Si mas.

For dizziness, do LI 11; it is great for that. I also use Three weights; they are especially helpful for older patients with dizziness. If you can, give him herbs. Here is what I often use: Tian ma 20%, Gou teng 20%, Ci shi 10%, Shi chang pu 10%, and 20% Ling gui zhu gan tang.

Another option is Ban xia bai zhu tian ma tang 50%, Ling gui zhu gan tang 25%, then add 25% of equal proportions of Tian ma, Gou teng, Ci shi, Shi chang pu, and Yuan zhi.

Either of those formulas is great. I just had two patients who had five treatments each who had dizzy wet/damp phlegm/blood stagnation tinnitus and Meniere's. I got no response with acupuncture—only about 15 percent relief. Then I put them on herbs; they were older, so they were on Medicare. They did not have enough money to come in all the time. They are great now!

For internal issues, herbs are usually best. For acupuncture points, you are doing the right thing. Local ear points, bleeding the ear apex (great work), upper leg points (nice), and Triple warmer and Large intestine points. Very nice.

It is not easy. Give it a few more times. Then you can have a talk with your patients. I would suggest you can get the dizziness to go away, but not the tinnitus. I bet you can reduce the ringing. I like to tell my patients that I bet I can reduce the ringing by 50–70 percent. But for the remainder, I am not sure.

My favorite points for Meniere's type dizziness are LI 11, Ling gu, Head three meetings 1010.01-5-6, GB 31, San cha san, the three weights 77.05-6-7. You could also try 77.27, the three lateral passes. We need to treat each patient according to the pattern they present.

Menstrual cycles and fertility timing

Hi Brad:

I recently viewed your webinar on fertility and have a question I can't seem to figure out.

Do you change the points at the various phases of a woman's menstrual cycle? Or just continue with one set of points each week regardless?

Brad: Yes, with acupuncture I do not separate it out per what week of the cycle it is. I do with herbs, for sure. But with acupuncture, I target the liver, the kidney, and whatever organ that is responsible. If it is stress, target the Shen.

I have my set points that I use for everybody for fertility that are about 50 percent of my treatment. Then, for the other 50 percent of the treatment, I pick points based on how the patient is presenting AT THAT POINT. So, yes, I guess you could say I choose points according to the week of the cycle. But I base my points off the patient, not the week of the cycle.

Mixing Chinese and Japanese, is that setting up for failure?

Hello Brad,

I was a participant in your Lotus Institute webinar given on the weekend of March 23rd of this year. I have been trying to incorporate your teachings into my practice since then.

Brad: It is easier than you think. Just do a little each day, and before you know it, you have it down.

Question: My question is this: I practice TCM style acupuncture using a mix of Chinese and Japanese styles. Am I setting myself up for failure by trying to just add some of the Dao Mas into my branch treatments rather than doing a full Tung treatment?

Brad: I do not think so; you just have to relax. Results are results. Who cares if it is Chinese, Tung, TCM, Five Element, or Japanese? Does the patient get better? Then keep using the same techniques. It just so happens that most of my techniques are Tung style acupuncture. I am only concerned about the results. If another technique gave me results, I would do that too.

So do not worry about what style you practice—just practice. You will see that the Chinese might say this, the Japanese say that, TCM says this, Tung says that, but in the end, it is not that much different. It is not as polar opposite as you think it is. It is all the same branch on the tree.

Question: I get to thinking about this in relation to the twenty-eight minutes it takes for the brain to "light up." If I leave the root treatment points in for fifteen minutes, then change the needles, have I disrupted the accumulated time so that the brain has to start the timer up again from zero?

Brad: Well, if you think you need to do a "root" and "branch" treatment, then do it if that is your style. They both work. I would argue that when you do Tung acupuncture, you are doing root and branch at the same time; that is why it is so powerful. I do not get caught up in that. I do the points, they work, people heal, and more people come in. But if you want to do a root treatment, then a branch treatment, that sounds great to me. I do not see the issue. I have no idea about "disrupted time" or this or that.

I would not worry so much about it. When it comes to pain, within two seconds the patient feels a difference. If it is internal, within two seconds the pulse will change to show you that you have fixed or are treating the root. But I treat my patients for thirty minutes. I do not care if it is one thirty-minute treatment, or three ten-minute treatments, or six five-minute treatments. I just treat them.

Question: Do the two different theory bases conflict?

Brad: Well, a theory is just that; it is a theory, not a scientific fact. So who cares if theories conflict? It is just two ways to look at the same thing.

Nocturnal enuresis in a ten-year-old boy

Hi Brad,

I took your Master Tung classes on line with Lotus. I have a question about treating nocturnal enuresis. Are there some Master Tung points or protocols you have had success with? My boy is ten and ready to move on from this. An acupuncturist I know said it was about calming the mind because an overactive child won't wake up. I think it is more than this though. He has a very active mind and takes longer to fall asleep. He has always had urgent urination. I did try a few bottles of Chai hu jia long gu mu li tang for him a few years ago.

Brad: Using Master Tung theory, we believe the spleen channel is the problem. The earth controls the water, so many spleen points will control the kidney issue. I usually do this treatment, and I help a lot of young boys with it.

125

According to Dr. Tung, it is usually caused by stress. Even Western doctors give kids an antidepressant for this.

For herbs, I usually use astringing things and calming things, like Wu wei zi, etc.

Acupuncture points:

Tung 77.18-19-21, 88.09-10-11, LU 7 (To fix the bottom, you must fix the top. The top organ is the lung; the bottom organ is kidney bladder.) Ren 24 (top of channel will fix bottom of channel), BL 2 bilateral. The face is the genital area, plus you get calming effects.

Tung 1010.05 area (Du 20 area), top balances bottom, Du balances Ren, and Du calms the shen and opens the mind.

Then add in the extra points.

I would probably use ear shen men, ear point zero, kidney point, lung point, and parasympathetic (calms down his nerves).

Parkinson's treatment

Hello Brad!

Thank you for the work you are doing! What would be your approach in treating Parkinson's? I am an L.Ac. and RN and have been diagnosed with Parkinson's for five years. (I am forty-nine now.)

Brad: I am sorry to hear that; let us see if we can figure something out.

Question: My tremor started in the left big toe, then it went to the left leg, then to the left arm. I am now on medications, so I am still able to practice medicine, but it is getting worse. Do you have any ideas?

Brad: Since you are an L.Ac. and an RN, I will tell you different things, because it is you, not your patient. We can be more aggressive. So let us get started.

First off, keep taking your medicine. Commit to your treatment, to yourself, for at least six months. Once you have that commitment, you will treat yourself—or have your friend treat you—two to three times a week for six months.

For herbs, Neuro Plus by Evergreen is awesome! I would strongly suggest that. Use about 70% that formula with 30% Circulation SJ, four grams twice a day, for six months.

I would STRONGLY suggest herbs with acupuncture. Do not do just acupuncture; do both!

Acupuncture

From a Tung perspective, we need to treat the liver and the tendons. The liver controls shaking and the tendons. We need to treat wind, which is weird and odd diseases, like Parkinson's, and we need to target blood circulation.

127

I would treat GB 31, LU 5, PC 3, Three meetings (Du 19-20-21) with Si shen cong, ST 36. I would mirror image the affected joint/limb. So, in your case, I would treat the left big toe and the left leg. I would stick to needling the bilateral big thumbs.

It is very interesting that the first metacarpal is the most innervated and therefore the highest neurological feedback to the mid-cortex of your brain. I would needle bilateral thumbs. This is Su Jok hand acupuncture, Master Tung image. Google Su Jok acupuncture.

Needle both thumbs, bilateral on the MIP and PIP joints, and put three needles down the thumb midline. The thumb here is your head, and the back of your thumb is your spine. It works great!

I would do the three upper yellows: tian huang, ming huang, qi huang. Again, Google the location; they are for the liver. The liver is for tendon shaking.

Also, the three weights will push blood in the head. That is very important for you and the three emperors (SP 6, 7 and 8.5). You can Google the location.

So that would be one treatment, the Master Tung, Five Element type of treatment.

The other treatment you should do would be the 12 Magical by Dr. Tan.

One arm: All yin jing wells
Other arm: LI 3, SI 3, TW 3
One leg: SP 6, LV 5, KD 7
Other leg: ST 36, GB 34, BL 40.

Alternate the limbs so it goes yin/yang, yin/yang.

Then I would bleed once every three weeks.

Bleed: Ear apex (either one), GV 14, 15, 16, 17, 18
Bleed: LI 1, PC 9, HT 9, LV 1, GB 44

I bet dollars to donuts, you will get results if you do that. I know it is a time commitment and a lot of work, but do that for six months and see how you feel. I would suggest you would feel great.

And I was just going over Parkinson's notes. For Master Tung points, I would say that from the list below, I would use some of the points and alternate between the others. Here are the numbers; just look up the locations.

Tung:
77.18-19-21
88.26-27
88.12-13-14
1010.01-05-06-18

I hope all that helps. Do not give up; you can find the answer.

Post-Herpetic Neuralgia

Hi Brad,

I have just enjoyed an ELotus talk you gave on Tung and TCM Points. Thank you so much! I am contacting you about two challenging patients. One is a 92-year-old woman with post-herpetic neuralgia on the right side of her face and scalp. She is in a constant state of pain, scoring 8 plus points on the pain scale. She describes it as burning and stinging pain, and she cannot touch it.

Do you have any suggestions? I have done a lot of the distal, ST and LV points, LI 4, and Battlefield acupuncture in her ears. This is a chronic issue for her, not new.

My second patient has very bad tinnitus, and I have had no success treating this in the past. He has worked in very noisy environments all his life. Is there help for someone like this?

Brad: For hearing problems, it is unlikely that acupuncture will be able to cure that. In my experience, it is 98 percent likely it is not treatable with acupuncture.

Auricular acupuncture seems to work well for tinnitus. That has been the only type that works in my experience.

For shingles, you can treat locally; that might work. But I usually do Gan men, 33.11, and put two or three needles in the opposite arm. Also, do the three lateral passes on the same leg, 77.27. That seems to work well. But for a ninety-two-year-old, it can be hard. I have treated some older people for that as well. Some of them even have twenty-thirty years of post-shingle pain. It is very hard, but worth a try.

You can also try doing the thigh on the same side and the opposite side. The points are 88.12-13-14, with 88.25 bilateral. See if that helps. You can also try 11.07 on the opposite side.

Quick Fix for Calming People

Dear Brad:

Very enjoyable preview this evening! I really look forward to trying out the headache protocol. :) I was wondering if you have a quick fix for calming people? For instance, to treat someone with ADHD-like symptoms.

It is almost as if the mind is always running, and she can't focus on one thing for very long. I work with someone like that, and I would just like to get her on my table and "shut her down" for fifteen minutes! Do you have any suggestions?

Brad: For a person at work, in your office, I would recommend:

An mian
Ear shen men
Ear point zero
Du20 or head three meetings Dao Ma
Yin tang (1010.08 Tung point, which is about .5 cun above yin tang.)

If you can do body points, I would recommend:

Tung 33.02 heart three needles, which is basically PC 4, 5, 7

GB 31, 88.25 is a great "chill out" point.

If it is due to liver stagnation, do 77.05-6-7, the three weights with wai gai san, the three lateral passes.

Liver anger 11.17 (somewhat painful, but great finger points for stress)
12 magical approach by Dr. Tan
Your old TCM four gates (I do not really like these, but I guess it works.)

Restless leg syndrome

Dear Brad,

Have you had any success treating restless leg syndrome?
I have had lousy luck with RLS. One of my patients uses a bar of Ivory soap at the foot of her bed under the fitted sheet. No clue why it works, but she says it does and can even tell when it falls off the bed or her husband moves it.

Brad: I have heard about the soap; my grandma told me about it. She is ninety-three! That is what they used in the Great Depression. Herbally, consider if she is drinking enough water and taking enough magnesium, calcium, and potassium.

Western doctors prescribe a drug that affects dopamine to calm it down, or opiates or sedatives. The same drugs they use for Parkinson's are used for restless leg syndrome.

In my experience, Yi gan san, which treats stress and increases dopamine production, the Gou teng.

Yi gan san + Gou teng + Flex SC (same as Zhi gan cao tang. Bai shao and zhi gan cao—it is an herbal Flexeril.

That seems to work great. You might add He huan pi, or Shi chang pu, Ban xia hou po tang—those herbs and formulas all make serotonin. Again, calming people down. If it is more neuro-degenerative, I like Enhance Memory and Neuro Plus by Evergreen. For normal, stressed-out Americans who cannot calm down and shake all night in bed, you can try: Yi gan san + Gou teng + Flex SC. This combination is great for about 75 percent of the overall formula. You can then add in any herbs that you think fit the pattern, or that you think the person really needs.

For acupuncture points:

Jue yin/Shao yang or Jue yue yang ming by Dr. Tan

It is TW 3-10, one arm, PC 7-3 other arm, one leg GB 41 and 34, other leg LV 3-8.
Or LI 1-4, one arm, PC 9-6 one arm
one leg L1-4, one leg ST 45-41
Add in Si shen cong, yin tang, ear shen men, ear point zero, an mian

If you do not like Tan style, then use the above points and add in GB 34, LI 4, LV 3, LV 8 SP 6 and GB 31 bilateral.

Severe Sciatica in Australia

Hi Brad:

I'm located in Australia. I heard about eLotus when I attended Dr Tan's seminar in Melbourne in 2012 and have been totally hooked on the website's educational content ever since. Love your videos. I try to access the live webinars, but our continental times are way out of sync. We have nothing that compares here.

I have a specific reason for emailing you, flattery aside. I have a client with severe sciatic pain. I have used the usual point combos for the condition, but sustained relief eludes.

In Dr Wei Chei Young's text under 'sciatica' he says, 'If sciatica is severe, use Qian Yin as a guide point.' I have checked everywhere and can't find any reference to this point or its location. Does it exist or was this a typo?

We have few chances to access teachers around the world, though this is slowly changing, as folks come to realize that Australia is actually inhabited by other than kangaroos.

Brad: Thank you for the e-mail.

Let us see, Qian yin, per Wei Chieh Young, and I am sorry, but I do not speak Chinese. Qian Yin refers to Master Tung's needling methods.

Master Tung was a quiet person. He did not talk much. Often he would respond to students' questions by saying, "Observe and think for yourself." This way of teaching allowed Dr. Young to think freely and forced him to study hard and develop his own theories. Dr. Young was an intelligent and diligent student of Master Tung's.

In 1971, he developed a powerful and effective technique named "Chien-Yin (Pulling & Guiding) Needling Technique." This technique is one of the so-called "Three Major Needling Techniques in Master Tung's Acupuncture." The other two are "Dong Qi (Activate Qi)" and "Dao Ma (Serial Needles)."

In 1973, Dr. Young developed "Zhang-Fu Bei tong (Organ Divergent Communications) theory," originating the idea from Nei Jing. This theory is one of the theories Dr. Young applied to explain Master Tung's Acupuncture. In 1975, Dr. Young published *Zhen Jiao Jing Wei* (*The Longitude and Latitude of Acupuncture and Moxibustion*), the first book ever documenting Master Tung's points with expanded theories and clinical experiences. Master Tung highly commended the work and gave his encouragement.

That is how I understand "qian yin." I do not know of a point named "qian yin," but that does not mean it does not exist; it might be outside my understanding.

For sciatica, I use the opposite side San Cha Yi, er san, with Ling gu, and SI 4. In addition, 33.12, Xin men, Gu ci Yi Er San, and then Pian Jian, TW 14 area (2-3-4 needles up there). (I would not do all of those, but at least two different images/areas.)

The points to treat on the same side, assuming it is on the bladder channel, are BL 65-62-60-40. That will usually nail it. Again, we do not need all of these, but at least the shu stream point.

On the head, 1010.25 (state waters point). I cannot remember the point number, but the point that you slide down to EOP (external occipital protuberance) in the back of the head? That is an awesome point.

You will need a lot of points for stubborn pain. You might need all of those, or at least fifty percent of those points.

I will come to Australia and teach you and all the kangaroos. Keep me in mind. :-)

Varicose Veins

Hi Brad,

I enjoy learning from your Lotus webinars. Thank you so much for sharing your wisdom!

I am very interested in any acupuncture, herbal, nutrition, and other recommendations you have for treating and preventing large varicose veins along the upper medial thigh. The veins are located in the Ming Huang area. There is also blood stagnation in the heart, liver, gall bladder, Heart 8 palm analysis locations and medial LU 10 metacarpal locations. I am reading and using James H. Maher's books: The Dao Ma Needling Technique & Neurology for point-location reference. Thanks in advance for taking the time to read my email.

Brad: Thank you so much! I am glad I can help.

There are a few things to consider. If the valves, the perforator valves, are broken, varicose veins can be very difficult to treat.

If the vein is stagnated and congested, that is easy to fix. However, if the valve is broken due to age, childbirth, gravity, or any other cause, you will be able to fix it, but it will always come back once you stop because the valve is broken. With that being said, here are some treatment options.

My favorite thing is to bleed first. But since you are in America, unless you and the patient know each other well, I would not do it. There would be a lot of blood.

For herbs, Circulation SJ is amazing! (Evergreen formula). I usually use Bu yang hu wu tang + Circulation SJ+ Si ni san + Mao dong qing.

Your goal with herbs is to move blood and get rid of the water. Water is 40 percent of blood, and too much water causes MORE stagnation and congestion. That is why I love Mao dong qing. I usually do 60 percent blood moving; 20 percent makes the heart beat more, and 20 percent drains the water/dries the damp. So you can put your formula together as you see fit.

Tung acupuncture points I use include:
The points 3 weights, 66.03-4, 4 flowers, 3 lateral passes, heart gate, 3 brachial ancestors. (I like this a lot not only for what it does, but also because it images the problem area perfectly.)

You can rotate in and/or exchange with these points:
Ling gu, Da bai, 88.01-2-3, 88.09-10-11, 33.07-08 and add in 88.12-13-14. (I think it is basically 6 up and 8.5 cun up on TW channel from the wrist crease; really it is .5 fen lateral, but it is close enough.)

I hope that helps. I would do acupuncture two times a week for two weeks along with herbs. Then treat one time a week for two weeks, then once a month to every two months so that you can keep an eye on it and recheck your herbal formula.

Question: Thanks again for your advice on the herbs and acupuncture. I really appreciate it.

The great saphenous vein valves are broken, a very large vein. There was physical trauma tearing the vein; there is blood stagnation. Because of this, would a distal point be better to blood let, such as LV 8? Or would you go farther distal like LV 3? Bloodletting channels is something new to me. We never practiced in college, only the ear apex, so it is interesting to see. I practice in Canada, which is similar to the USA in regards to bloodletting.

I will work with the herbs and acupuncture and see how it goes. Thanks for sharing, and if you have any more info on treating veins I am very interested.

Brad: I would bleed locally in this case, though I usually do not.

Images

We have compiled images, mirrors, and pictures of relationships for your reference. By no means is this an "exhaustive" list of all the images, mirrors, and relationships. We have included these images to help the reader "see" some examples of the theories discussed in this book.

Please use this list and educational format to help the reader start to see how the "lungs are imaged on the arm" or the "heart is imaged on the leg." Hopefully, you can or will start to see the "twelve segments" and see the "groin imaged on the hands, shoulders, or face."

Throughout this book, we have referenced many Master Tung points. We have included some of these points for a simple understanding of "where" the points are. This is not meant to be a point-location book.

The images that are used are not specific enough to be used "solely" as your identifying marks for correct point placement. These images, though correct in location, are mostly for the reader to have a "visual" of where the points are versus just a "verbal" of where they are. Please use other resources for precise locations of these points. It is best to use Master Tung books, or classes, for the *exact* locations of the points in question.

Move out of your comfort zone. You can only grow if you are willing to feel awkward and uncomfortable when you try something new.

Brian Tracy

CHAPTER 6

ACUPUNCTURE MERIDIAN IMAGES

In order to use the Master Tung or the balance system correctly, you will need to remember the path of the meridian. We have included the meridians as well as the tendon meridians.

The meridian pathways and sinew channels are referenced from the *Manual of Acupuncture* by Peter Deadman and Mazin Al-Khafaji, with Kevin Baker.

We list the meridians alphabetically, and we reference the Chinese pin yin names for the Ren and Du meridians throughout the book.

Bladder, Urinary Bladder	BL
Du, Governing	Du
Gall Bladder	GB
Heart	HT
Kidney	KI
Large Intestine	LI
Liver	LV
Lungs	LU
Pericardium	PC
Ren, Conception	Ren
San Jiao, Triple Warmer	SJ, or TW
Small Intestine	SI
Spleen	SP
Stomach	ST

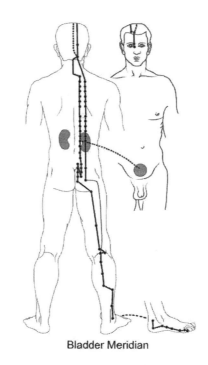

Bladder Meridian

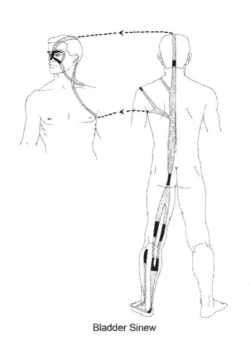

Bladder Sinew

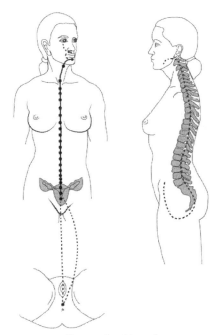

Conception Vessel

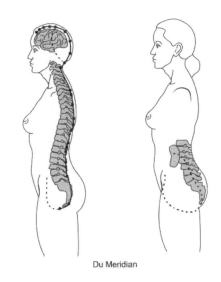

Du Meridian

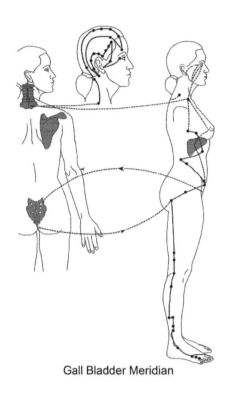

Gall Bladder Meridian

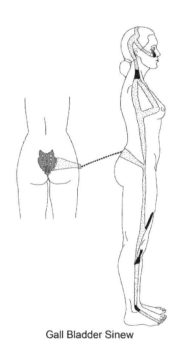

Gall Bladder Sinew

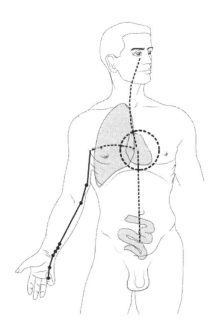

Heart Meridian

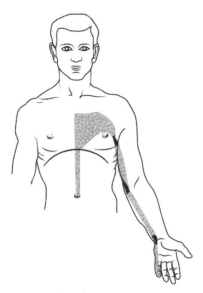

Heart Sinew

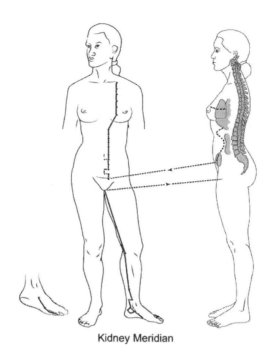

Kidney Meridian

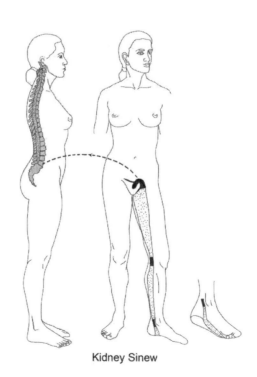

Kidney Sinew

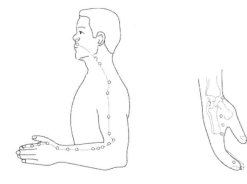

Large Intestine Meridian

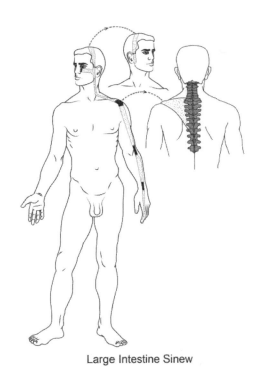

Large Intestine Sinew

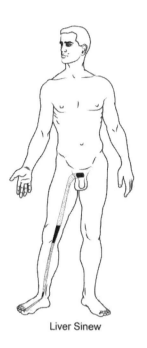

Liver Sinew

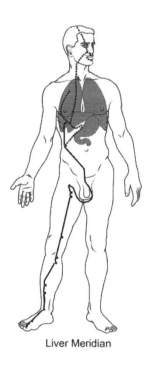

Liver Meridian

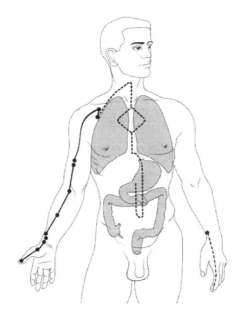

Lung Meridian

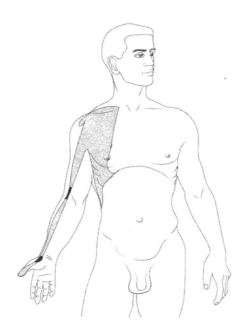

Lung Sinew

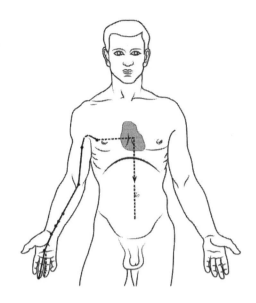

Pericardium Meridian

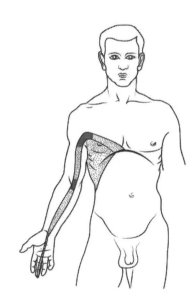

Pericardium Sinew

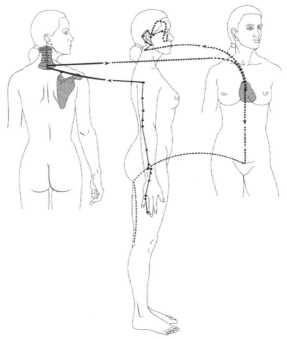

San Jiao Meridian

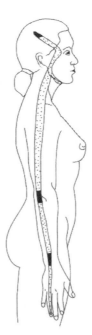

San Jiao Sinew

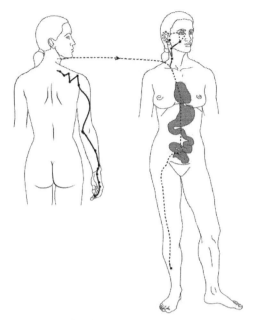

Small Intestine Meridian

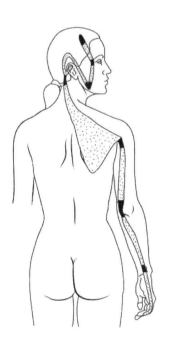

Small Intestine Sinew

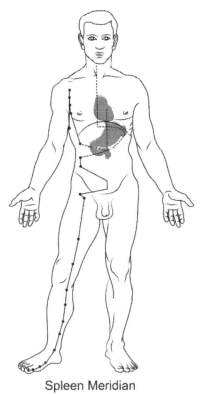

Spleen Meridian

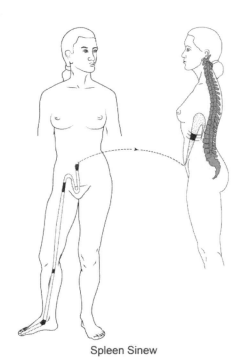

Spleen Sinew

151

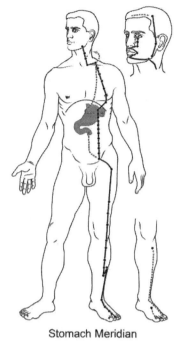

Stomach Meridian

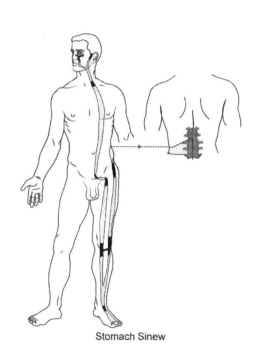

Stomach Sinew

CHAPTER 7

IMAGING TABLES

Imaging limbs to head

Upper limb	Head	Lower limb
Shoulder joint	Top of head	Hip joint
Upper arm	Forehead	Upper leg
Elbow	Eye, ear	Knee
Forearm	Nose level	Lower leg
Wrist and hand	Mouth level	Ankle and foot
Fingers	Chin level	Toes

Imaging limbs to head and trunk

Upper limb	Head and trunk image	Lower limb
Top of shoulder	Top of head	Top of hip
Shoulder	Neck, jaw, base of skull	Hip joint
Upper arm	Chest, mid-upper back	Upper leg
Elbow	Xiphoid process, diaphragm	Knee
Forearm	Lower abs, lower back	Lower leg
Wrist	Pubic symphysis, bladder, sacrum	Ankle
Hand	Genitals, coccyx, lower sacrum	Foot
Finger	Testicles, anus	Toe

Reverse imaging: limbs to head

Upper limb	Head	Lower limb
Fingers	Top of head	Toes
Wrist and hand	Between top of head and forehead	Ankle and foot
Forearm	Forehead	Lower leg
Elbow	Eye, ear	Knee
Upper arm	Nose level	Upper leg
Shoulder	Mouth level	Hip
Shoulder joint	Chin level	Hip joint

Reverse imaging: limbs to head and trunk

Upper limb	Head and trunk image	Lower limb
Finger	Top of head	Toe
Hand	Head, base of skull	Foot
Wrist	Neck	Ankle
Forearm	Chest, mid and upper back	Lower leg
Elbow	Xiphoid process, diaphragm	Knee
Upper arm	Lower abdominal muscles, lower back	Upper leg
Shoulder	Sacrum, genitals, coccyx	Hip joint
Top of shoulder	Testicles, anus	Top of hip

Chapter 8

Tung Acupuncture Point Illustrations

1010.08
1010.21-22
1010.25
11.01-2-3-4
11.09-11.13
11.17
22.01-2
22.04-5
33.06-7
33.08-09
44.02-3-4
44.06, 44.10-11-12
55.02 a 4 point unit /55.06
66.03-4, 5/66.06-7 , 8, 9
66.10-11-12
77.01-2-3
77.08, 09
77.17-18-19-20-21 , 17
77.24
77.26, 3 point unit
77.27, 3 point unit
88.01-2-3
88.25
San Cha san.---A 02,

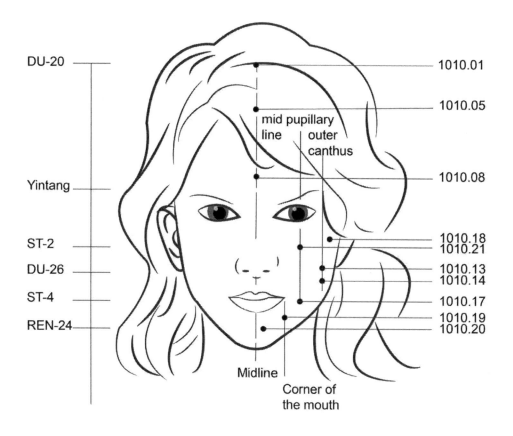

DU-20 ———————————————— 1010.01

—————————————— 1010.05

mid pupillary
line   outer
canthus

Yintang ————— 1010.08

ST-2 ————— 1010.18
1010.21

DU-26 ————— 1010.13
1010.14

ST-4 ————— 1010.17

REN-24 ————— 1010.19
1010.20

Midline

Corner of
the mouth

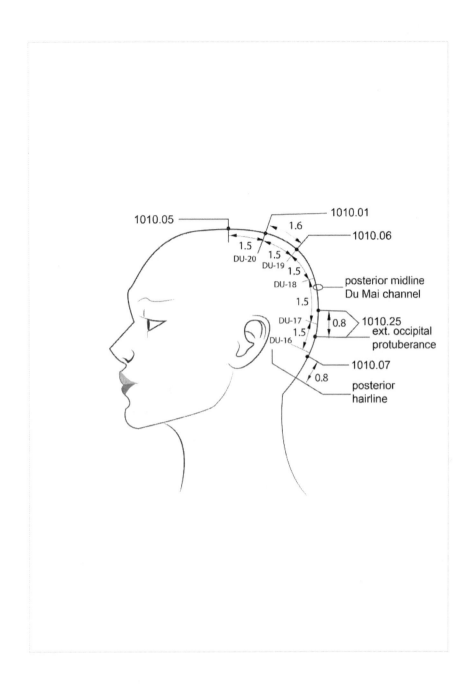

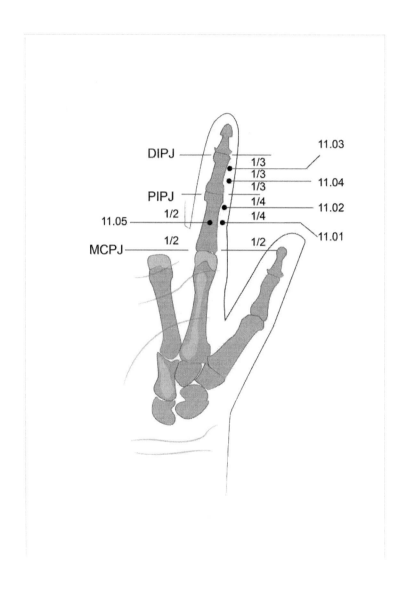

DIPJ

1/3   11.03

1/3

1/3   11.04

PIPJ

1/4   11.02

1/2

11.05   1/4   11.01

MCPJ   1/2   1/2

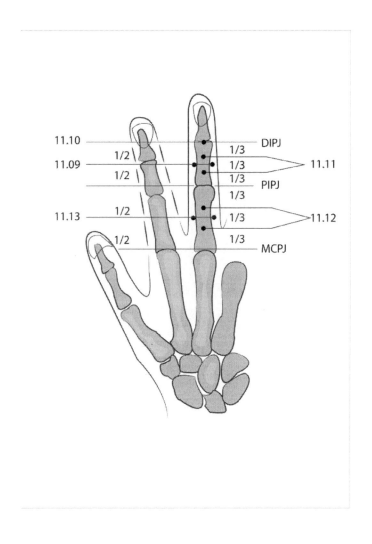

11.10

1/2

11.09

1/2

11.13

1/2

1/2

DIPJ

1/3

1/3

1/3

1/3

PIPJ

1/3

1/3

1/3

MCPJ

11.11

11.12

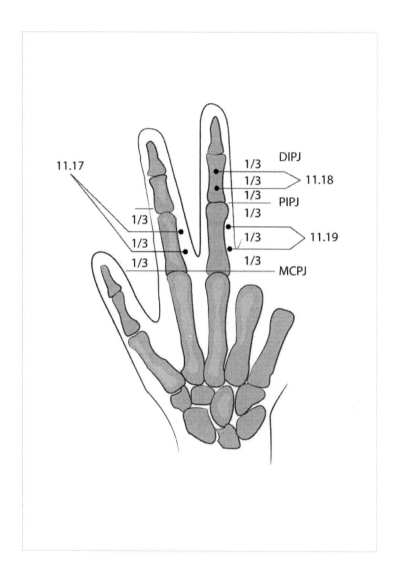

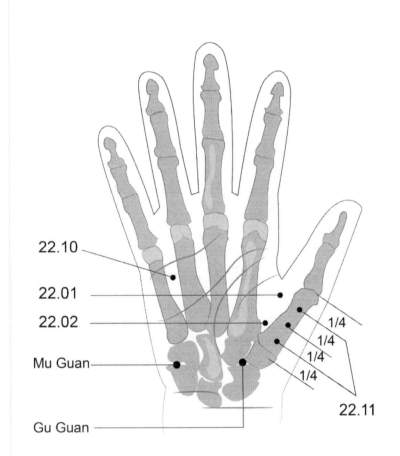

22.10

22.01

22.02

Mu Guan

Gu Guan

1/4

1/4

1/4

1/4

22.11

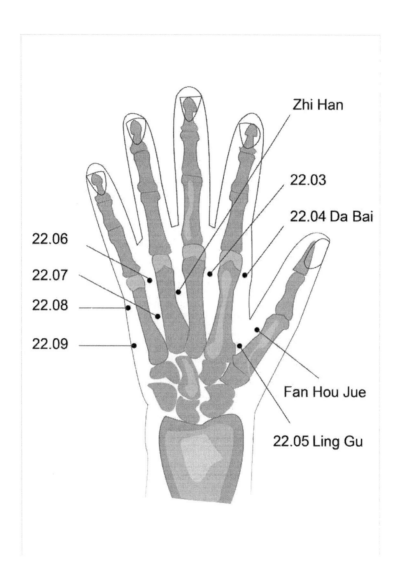

Zhi Han

22.03

22.04 Da Bai

22.06

22.07

22.08

22.09

Fan Hou Jue

22.05 Ling Gu

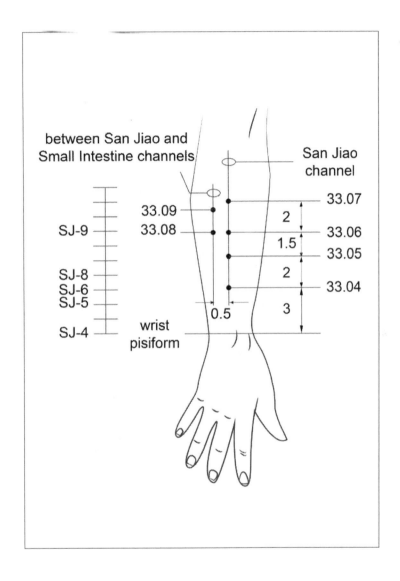

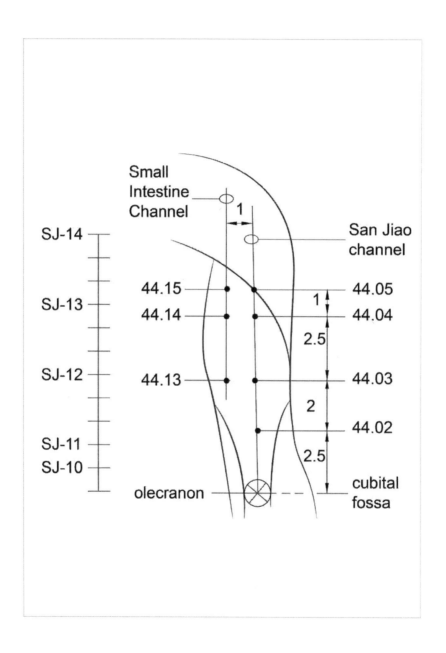

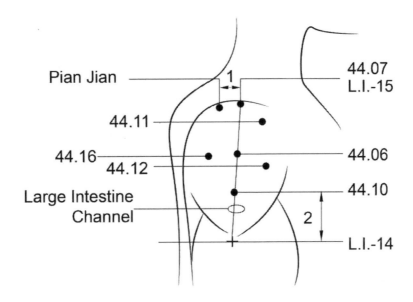

Pian Jian

44.11

44.16
44.12

Large Intestine
Channel

44.07
L.I.-15

44.06

44.10

L.I.-14

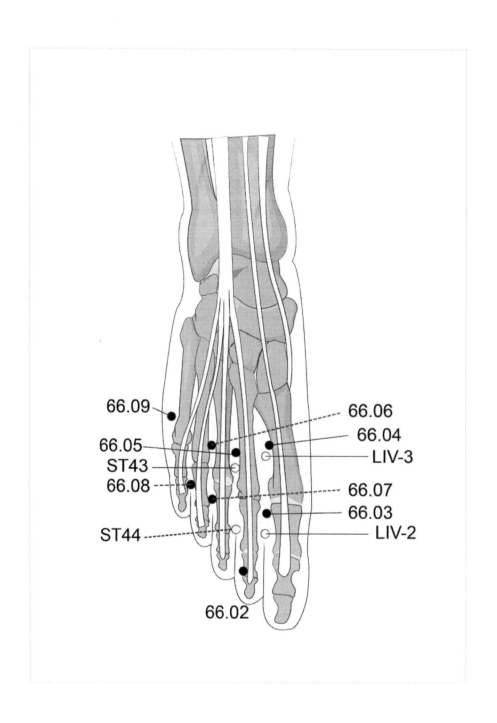

66.09

66.06

66.05
66.04

ST43
LIV-3

66.08
66.07

66.03

ST44
LIV-2

66.02

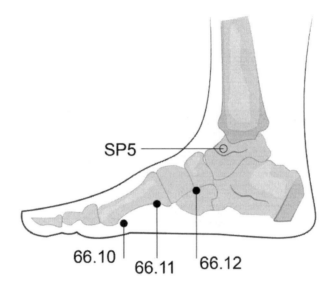

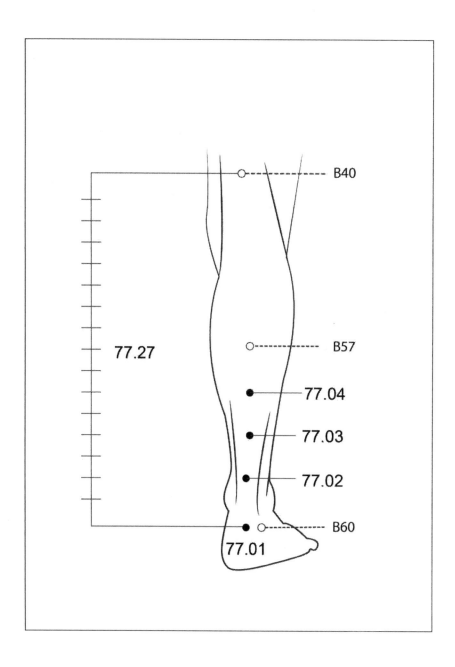

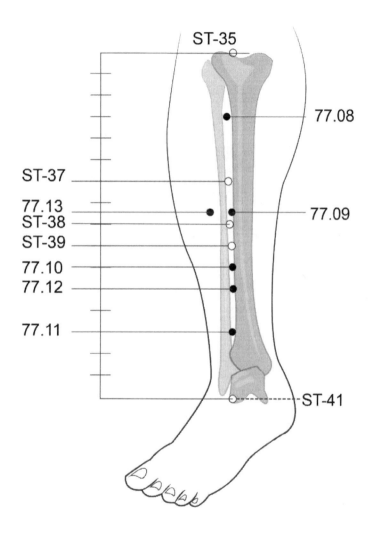

169

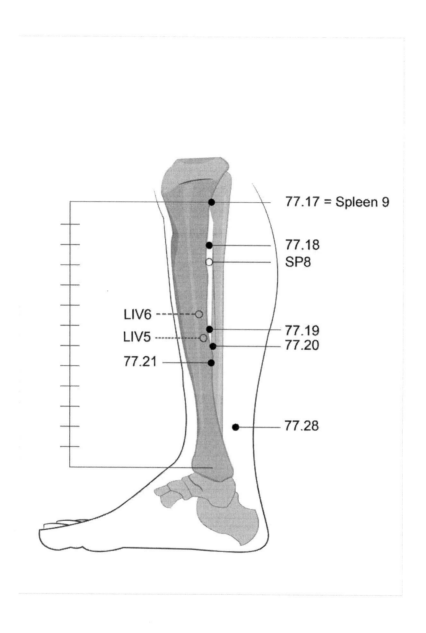

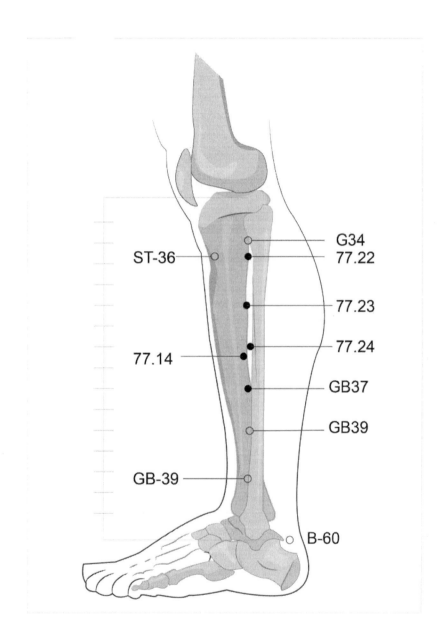

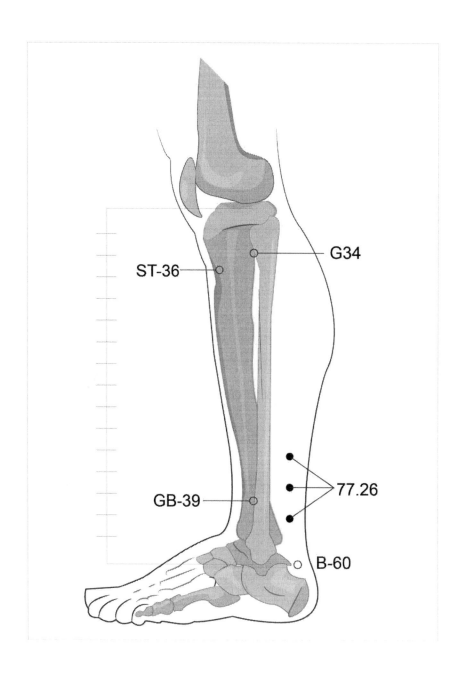

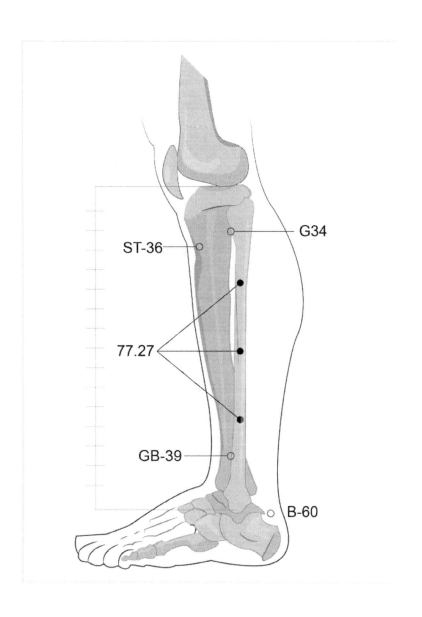

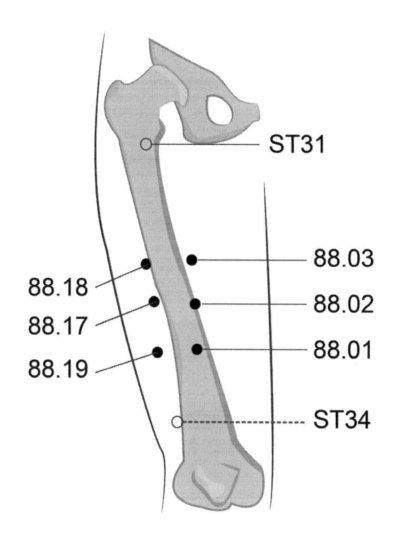

ST31

88.18

88.17

88.19

88.03

88.02

88.01

ST34

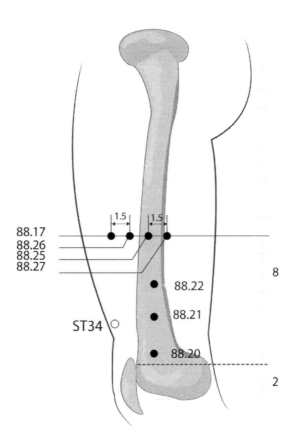

88.17
88.26
88.25
88.27

1.5 1.5

88.22

88.21

88.20

ST34

8

2

175

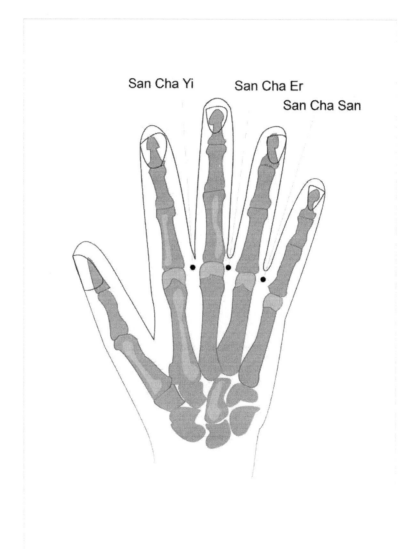

San Cha Yi   San Cha Er
San Cha San

CHAPTER 9

ANATOMY REFERENCES – MUSCLES AND BONES

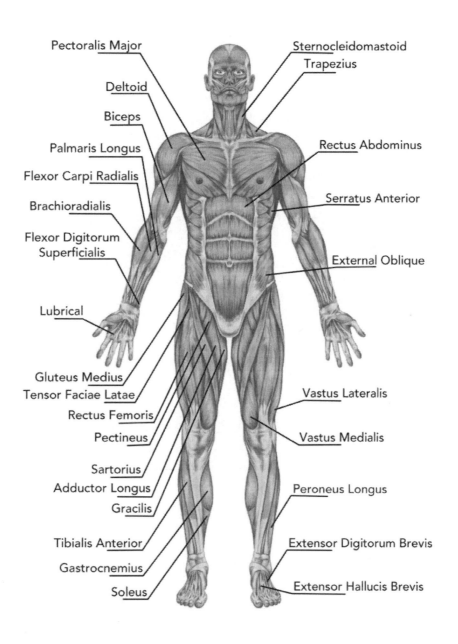

Pectoralis Major

Deltoid

Biceps

Palmaris Longus

Flexor Carpi Radialis

Brachioradialis

Flexor Digitorum
Superficialis

Lubrical

Gluteus Medius
Tensor Faciae Latae

Rectus Femoris

Pectineus

Sartorius

Adductor Longus

Gracilis

Tibialis Anterior

Gastrocnemius

Soleus

Sternocleidomastoid
Trapezius

Rectus Abdominus

Serratus Anterior

External Oblique

Vastus Lateralis

Vastus Medialis

Peroneus Longus

Extensor Digitorum Brevis

Extensor Hallucis Brevis

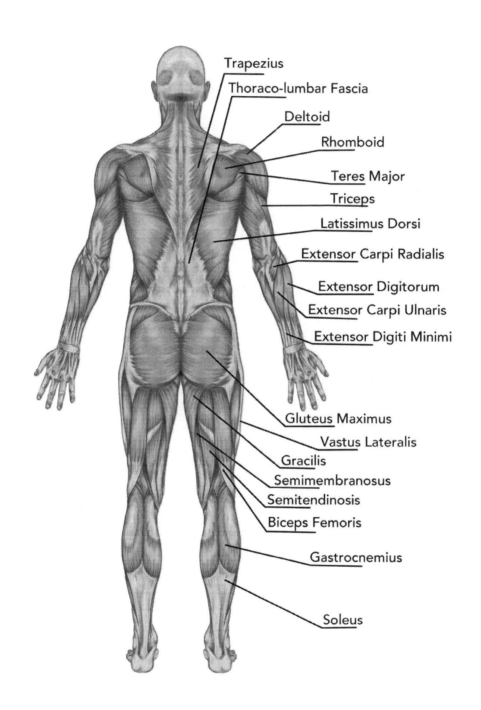

Trapezius

Thoraco-lumbar Fascia

Deltoid

Rhomboid

Teres Major

Triceps

Latissimus Dorsi

Extensor Carpi Radialis

Extensor Digitorum

Extensor Carpi Ulnaris

Extensor Digiti Minimi

Gluteus Maximus

Vastus Lateralis

Gracilis

Semimembranosus

Semitendinosis

Biceps Femoris

Gastrocnemius

Soleus

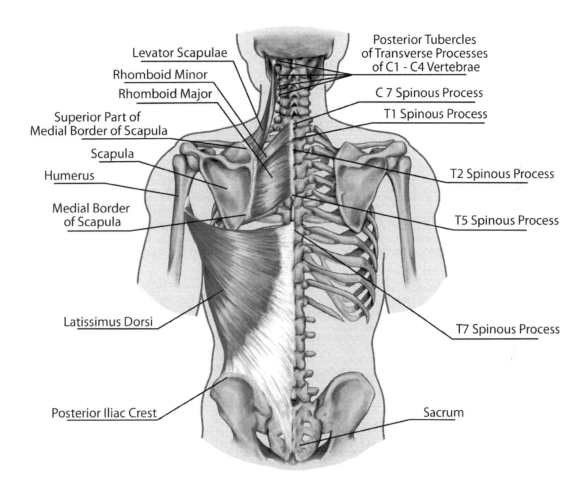

Levator Scapulae

Rhomboid Minor

Rhomboid Major

Superior Part of
Medial Border of Scapula

Scapula

Humerus

Medial Border
of Scapula

Latissimus Dorsi

Posterior Iliac Crest

Posterior Tubercles
of Transverse Processes
of C1 - C4 Vertebrae

C 7 Spinous Process

T1 Spinous Process

T2 Spinous Process

T5 Spinous Process

T7 Spinous Process

Sacrum

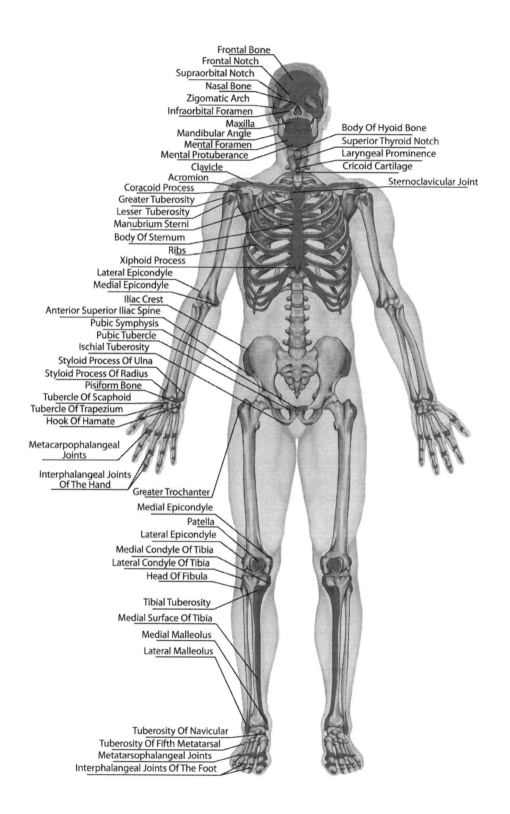

Frontal Bone
Frontal Notch
Supraorbital Notch
Nasal Bone
Zigomatic Arch
Infraorbital Foramen
Maxilla
Mandibular Angle
Mental Foramen
Mental Protuberance
Clavicle
Acromion
Coracoid Process
Greater Tuberosity
Lesser Tuberosity
Manubrium Sterni
Body Of Sternum
Ribs
Xiphoid Process
Lateral Epicondyle
Medial Epicondyle
Iliac Crest
Anterior Superior Iliac Spine
Pubic Symphysis
Pubic Tubercle
Ischial Tuberosity
Styloid Process Of Ulna
Styloid Process Of Radius
Pisiform Bone
Tubercle Of Scaphoid
Tubercle Of Trapezium
Hook Of Hamate
Metacarpophalangeal Joints
Interphalangeal Joints Of The Hand
Greater Trochanter
Medial Epicondyle
Patella
Lateral Epicondyle
Medial Condyle Of Tibia
Lateral Condyle Of Tibia
Head Of Fibula
Tibial Tuberosity
Medial Surface Of Tibia
Medial Malleolus
Lateral Malleolus
Tuberosity Of Navicular
Tuberosity Of Fifth Metatarsal
Metatarsophalangeal Joints
Interphalangeal Joints Of The Foot

Body Of Hyoid Bone
Superior Thyroid Notch
Laryngeal Prominence
Cricoid Cartilage
Sternoclavicular Joint

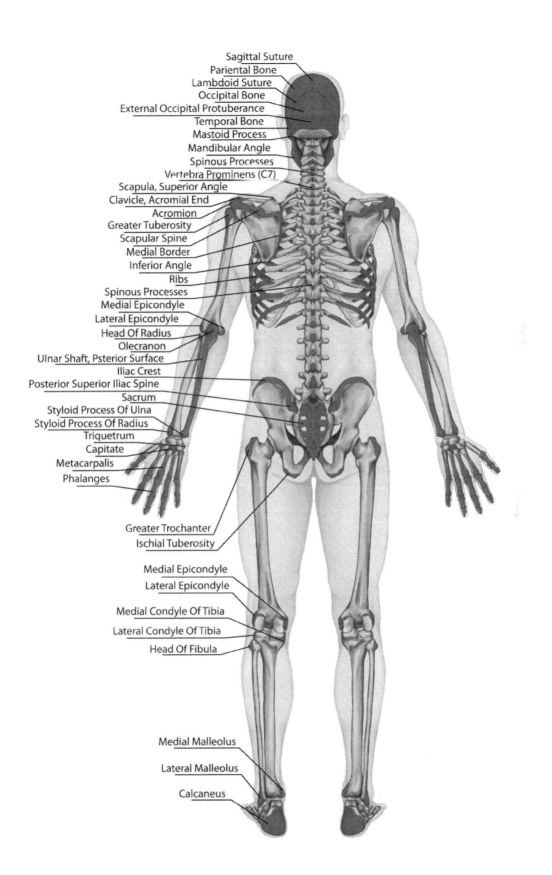

Sagittal Suture
Pariental Bone
Lambdoid Suture
Occipital Bone
External Occipital Protuberance
Temporal Bone
Mastoid Process
Mandibular Angle
Spinous Processes
Vertebra Prominens (C7)
Scapula, Superior Angle
Clavicle, Acromial End
Acromion
Greater Tuberosity
Scapular Spine
Medial Border
Inferior Angle
Ribs
Spinous Processes
Medial Epicondyle
Lateral Epicondyle
Head Of Radius
Olecranon
Ulnar Shaft, Psterior Surface
Iliac Crest
Posterior Superior Iliac Spine
Sacrum
Styloid Process Of Ulna
Styloid Process Of Radius
Triquetrum
Capitate
Metacarpalis
Phalanges

Greater Trochanter
Ischial Tuberosity

Medial Epicondyle
Lateral Epicondyle

Medial Condyle Of Tibia
Lateral Condyle Of Tibia
Head Of Fibula

Medial Malleolus

Lateral Malleolus

Calcaneus

The majority of men meet with failure because of their lack of persistence in creating new plans to take the place of those that fail.

Napoleon Hill

CHAPTER 10

CORRESPONDENCE IMAGES

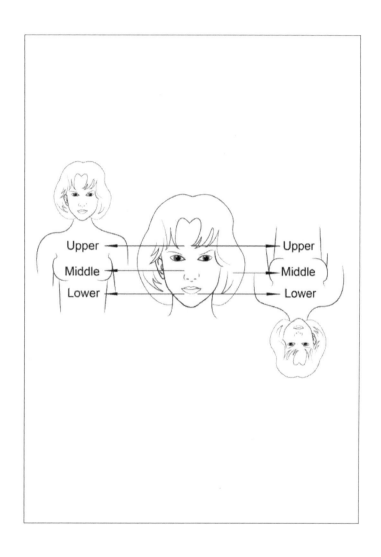

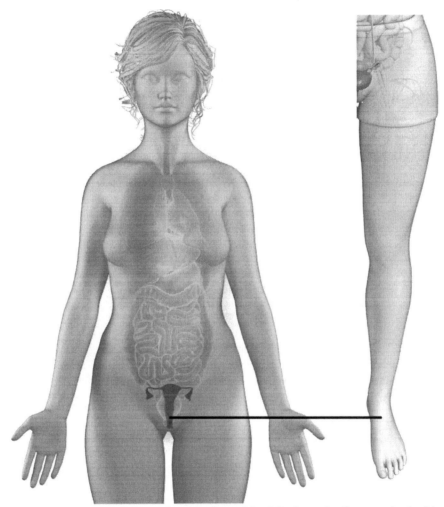

There are many points on the hands and feet that are for "gynecological issues" **66.13-14-15, 66.01, 55.01,** *and* **66.05** *are indicated for the uterus. Depending on your particular medical complaint, certain points are used versus the other points. One thing they have in common is the "correct image" The foot is a great image of the "Full Torso on the Full limb", in this case the leg. One can see the foot in this case represents the lower gynecological area.*

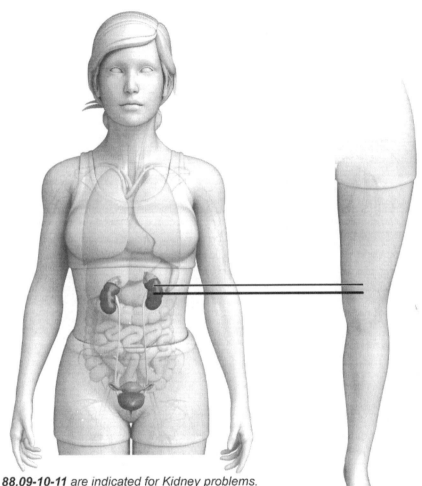

88.09-10-11 are indicated for Kidney problems.
*The Earth/Spleen controls the Water/Kidney. The image of this
is the "Full Leg on the Full Torso." The first point is at the
superior, medial border of the patella, on the Spleen channel.
The next point 88.10 is 2 cun proximal, and then 88.11 is 2 cun
more proximal. The kidneys are on the same level as these points.
These 3 points cover the superior, middle and inferior aspects of the kidney.*

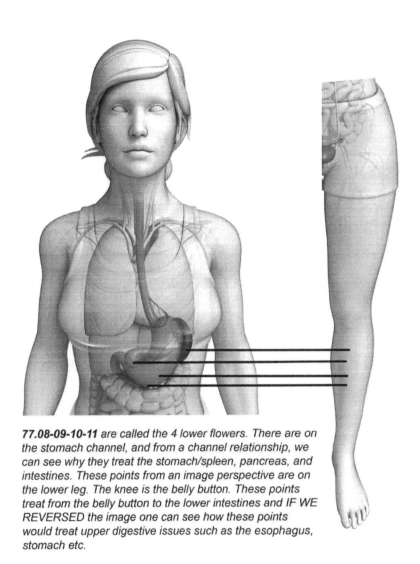

77.08-09-10-11 *are called the 4 lower flowers. There are on the stomach channel, and from a channel relationship, we can see why they treat the stomach/spleen, pancreas, and intestines. These points from an image perspective are on the lower leg. The knee is the belly button. These points treat from the belly button to the lower intestines and IF WE REVERSED the image one can see how these points would treat upper digestive issues such as the esophagus, stomach etc.*

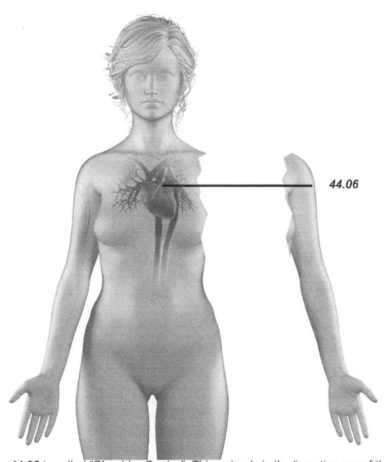

44.06 is called "Shoulder Center". This not only is the "reaction are of the cardiac nerve" it is also at the same level as the heart. This is not an image of the torso on the limb, this image is merely an image of "observance". Where is the heart if we were to put it on the arm? The point 44.06 is exactly where the heart is. Fabulous point for heart conditions

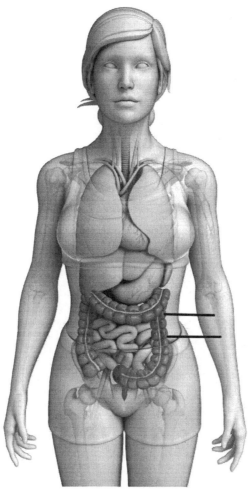

*Shou Wu Jin and Shou Qin Jin are named **33.08-09**. The are INBETWEEN the TW and SI channels. In the Master Tung system many points are in-between channels. These points are located 6.5 and 8 cun proximal from the wrist crease, .5 cun lateral to the TW channel. When points are in-between channels they treat both channels. In this case, **33.08-09** are both the TW and SI and thus treat all those relationships of the TW and SI. Not only from an image perspective but also all the channels that the TW and SI treat. We can easily see why **33.08-09** treat so many digestive problems.*

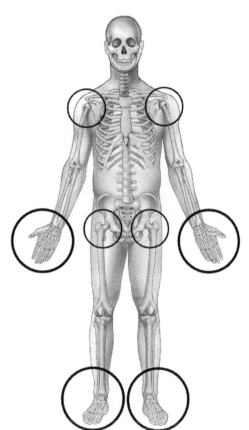

This images is a "homologous" relationship. The hip and shoulders look just alike, as do the feet and hands. What other bones do you see that look just like each other?

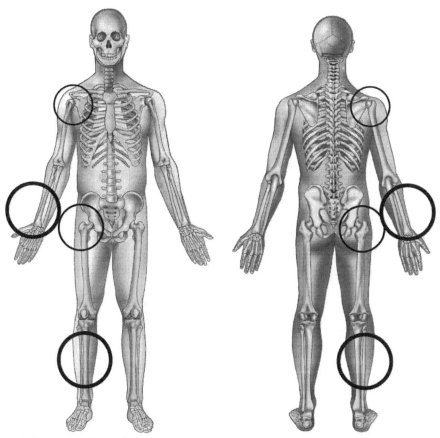

This is another "Homologous" relationship. The lower leg bones look just like the lower arm bones. The scapula and posterior shoulder look like the posterior hip, femur and sacrum. The lateral side of the sacrum is the lateral side of the scapula. The L5/S1 joint is the posterior shoulder joint, where the scapula meets the humerus much like where SI 10 is. The top of pelvic girdle is the spine of scapula. Can you see other homologous relationships?

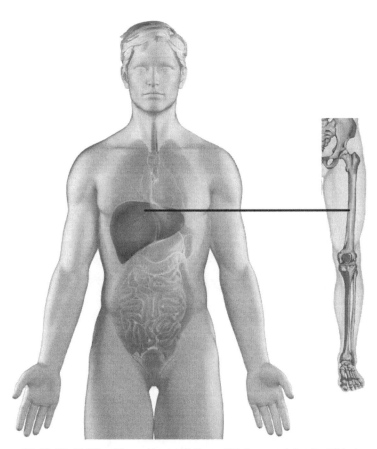

88.12-13-14 *"The Three Upper Yellows." Yellow explains that it helps with the Liver. Yellow is typically the color a person will turn when his liver is malfunctioning. Locate this point by finding **GB 31** or **88.25**. Take that EXACT POINT, and transfer that point to the liver channel. This is **88.12, 88.13** and **88.14** are above and below **88.12** by 3 cun a piece respectively. This is an image of the "Full torso on the Full Leg". The mid-thigh and mid abdomen, the liver, are on the same level.*

Never, never, never give up.

Winston Churchill

Resources

Brad can be reached at:

masteringtungacupuncture@yahoo.com
www.sthelensacupuncturist.com
www.masteringtungacupuncture.com

Check out our website for:

- New book news
- Training sessions with Brad – Seminars coming in 2016

Please sign up for our mailing list to be notified of new books and training sessions.

Evergreen Herbs & Medical Supplies, LLC

17431 East Gale Ave
City of Industry, CA 91748

Tel: 626-810-5530   Toll-Free Tel: 866-473-3697 (GREEN97)
Fax: 626-810-5534   Toll-Free Fax: 866-473-3698 (GREEN98)

Email: sales@evherbs.com

www.elotus.org and www.evherbs.com

Elotus is the Lotus Institute of Integrative Medicine. They offer hundreds of hours of training in acupuncture and all aspects of Chinese medicine.

Evergreen and Elotus have been at the forefront of bringing education and enlightenment to our industry for a long time. Evergreen provides many valuable resources for information on Chinese medicine. Elotus is at the forefront of online education for acupuncturists. Acupuncturists all over the world benefit from their dedication to our profession. Without their support, many of us, including myself, would be lost and struggling in our profession. I appreciate and admire both of these companies.

The Crane Herb Companies

Crane Herb Company, Inc.
745 Falmouth Road
Mashpee, MA 02649

Tel: 508-539-1700

info@craneherb.com

www.craneherb.com

Crane-West Herb Pharmacy, Inc.
515 South Main St.
Sebastopol, CA 95472

Tel: 707-823-5691

crane-west@craneherb.com

Crane Herbs provides over thirty-eight brands of Chinese herbs, as of this writing. They also offer ten brands of acupuncture needles. They carry many types of acupuncture supplies. They offer drop shipping direct to your patient or family member via their patient pharmacy. They also offer a custom pharmacy.

Please note that Crane Herb Company ONLY sells to state-licensed and nationally certified Chinese medicine practitioners. They do not sell to the public.

References

Practical Atlas of Tung's Acupuncture – 2014
Henry McCann (Author) and Hans-Georg Ross (Author)

Acupuncture 1, 2, 3
Dr. Tan's Strategy of 12 Magical Points
Twelve & Twelve in Acupuncture
Twenty-Four More in Acupuncture
Richard Teh-Fu Tan and Stephen Rush, OMD, LAc.

Lectures on Tung's Acupuncture – Points Study, 2008
Tung's Acupuncture, 2005
Lectures on Tung's Acupuncture Therapeutic System, 2008
Dr. Wei Chieh Young

Introduction to Tung's Acupuncture – 2014
Dr. Chuan-Min Wang DC LAc (Author), Steven Vasilakis LAc (Editor)

Advanced Tung Style Acupuncture: The Dao Ma Needling Technique of Master Tung Ching Chang
James H. Maher

Master Tung's Acupuncture: An Ancient Alternative Style in Modern Clinical Practice, Oct 1992
Miriam Lee

Made in the USA
Middletown, DE
14 June 2015